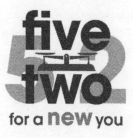

five 52 two

for a **new** you

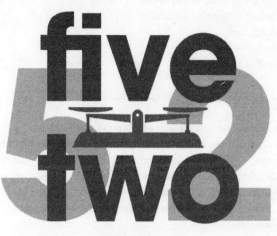

five two
52

for a new you

The fast formula for a happier, healthier life

Janet Menzies

Michael O'Mara Books Limited

First published in Great Britain in 2013 by
Michael O'Mara Books Limited
9 Lion Yard
Tremadoc Road
London SW4 7NQ

A CIP catalogue record for this book is available from the British
Library.

Papers used by Michael O'Mara Books Limited are natural,
recyclable products made from wood grown in sustainable
forests. The manufacturing processes conform to the
environmental regulations of the country of origin.

ISBN: 978-1-78243-218-0 in paperback print format
ISBN: 978-1-78243-235-7 in ebook format

1 2 3 4 5 6 7 8 9 10

Designed and typeset by K.DESIGN, Winscombe, Somerset

Printed and bound by CPI Group (UK) Ltd, Croydon, CR0 4YY

www.mombooks.com

Contents

Acknowledgements

A massive thank you goes out to my family and friends who were all so patient and tolerant while I was obsessing on this book. Lisa Sewards gave me massive support and help, along with Hugh Morris, Nathan Champ and Sally Monkhouse. Some of you even volunteered to help with the research by being 'test pilots' and 'air controllers'. To avoid potential embarrassment I haven't used your names – but you know who you are, so thank you very much!

Thank you also to my agent, James Wills, for teaming me up with Michael O'Mara Books, and to Louise Dixon, Gabriella Nemeth, Emily Banyard and the team at Michael O'Mara Books.

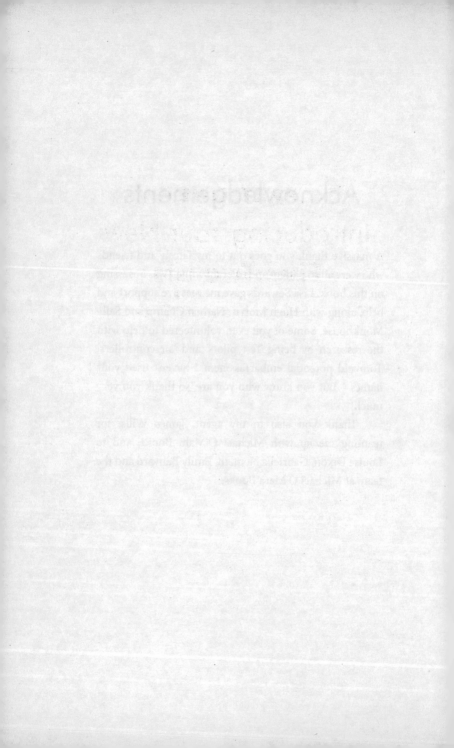

PART ONE
Introducing Your New **Five:Two** Life

What **Five:Two** Can Do For You

Sometimes your life feels like a balancing act. Now here's a method to put your life in balance. *Five:Two For a New You* can teach you how to improve your figure and fitness, how to make your relationships less stressful, and even how to put the life back into your working life. You will learn methods to help organize many different aspects of life so that you can achieve the goals you want. You can use the regime to beat the signs of ageing and bring some relaxation into even the most frantic schedule.

We all know that balance is important, but modern life can make it impossible to keep that balance. Twenty-four/seven social media, advertising pressure, work demands, and constant juggling, all mean that we lose sight of the simple basics to enjoy life. This book gives you the techniques to get back in control, without having to give up the things you enjoy. Once you get used to the method, you can apply it to anything in your life that you want to regain control of. Instead of all-or-nothing rules that can't be kept, you will learn the arts of balance and compromise that will last you for ever.

> **Five:Two** turns 'I ought to' into 'I want to'
>
> **Two** of great is worth **Five** of OK
>
> **Five:Two** makes 'I should' into 'I will'

Wonky wheels?

If your life is out of balance it's like trying to get the supermarket shop done when you've grabbed a trolley with a wonky wheel. You know what happens – the thing has a mind of its own and you keep crashing into the shelf stacks. It's a huge struggle to get it going straight, and then that wonky wheel keeps dragging it off-course. And as you get more stuff in the trolley the problem gets worse and worse. By the time you're back out in the car park, you're shattered from trying to push against that wonky wheel all the time. The whole thing is exhausting.

It's just the same if your life has a 'wonky wheel'. You think you're back on track for a while, but then more stuff is going on in your life – just like your supermarket trolley getting fuller – and pretty soon the wonky wheel underneath is pulling you back off-course again. Like trying to go up and down the aisles, even day-to-day life becomes a huge struggle when things are out of balance.

Get your trolley back on track

But the original idea of supermarket trolleys was to make shopping easier. When you happen to pick a brand-new trolley with smooth wheels, you whisk round the aisles in no time. Even when you have a really big weekly shop and there are loads of things in your trolley, the wheels are running so well that you've soon got all the bags in the boot of the car with a minimum of effort. It will be just the same when you learn the techniques in this book. No more wonky wheels – every day will be a new trolley day. Even if your life is really busy – just like a very full supermarket trolley – you will be able to keep all those different things in balance, so that you can cope comfortably without feeling you are being dragged in different directions.

The balanced life

Just imagine waking up in the morning with a sense that you are looking forward to the day, even if you know you've got a really busy time ahead of you. You may have a dozen different things that need to be done, but with these balance methods, you are going to be equal to all of them. It will put an end to that feeling that things are getting out of hand, because if things are in balance, they can't get on top of you.

All the different formulas are here to help you with a load of different problems you may be worried about.

The formulas act like recipes, giving you a step-by-step approach to solving your anxieties. It's all about finding the right solution for your particular issue.

Waking up to a new you

You will be amazed at the change in your life once you have started using the new formulas. Remember the difference when you swap that wonky trolley for a new one? Without the strain of pushing the wonky trolley, suddenly you will find you have mounds more energy. Things that seemed almost impossibly difficult will feel quite achievable.

When I made this programme a regular, permanent part of my life, I couldn't believe how different I felt about things. The first thing I noticed was how much less physically tired I was. This surprised me because I didn't think that my issues were physical ones. But the stress of being out of balance all the time was actually having a physical impact on fatigue and lost sleep. Some friends said I actually looked like I had grown an inch! I think this was because I really did feel like a wonky trolley, all twisted out of shape with worry. When I fixed that wonky wheel, it felt like I was able to stand up taller – it had genuinely taken a weight off my shoulders.

I noticed more changes. After I had been using this method for a while, and had got the hang of how to apply it in different situations, I began to feel a really unusual thing.

Problems – even quite stressful ones – hardly worried me at all. It really was an out-of-the-ordinary feeling. If a difficult situation, or even a real crisis, blew up at home, or about work, or with family and friends, I began to react in a way that was much more calm and confident. I would say to myself: 'Hmm, this is a tricky one, but this technique will have the answer. If I just give myself a while to work out how I can apply it, I will find a solution.'

Feeling positive – permanently

Then gradually, this more positive attitude towards life issues developed into being my normal mindset. As a writer, I suppose I'm naturally a creative person, and I think what must have happened with the help of this method was that a lot of my energy was freed up to use towards the fun, creative, happy aspects of life, rather than being wasted on worrying about all those out-of-balance issues. I found my enjoyment of life sky-rocketed. Even the most simple of things became really noticeable pleasures. Taking time to home-cook a lovely meal. Sitting down for an hour with a good book. Walking the dogs. I know they are only little things, but I suddenly found I was enjoying them as much as a foreign holiday. I began to look forward to every day – even the ones that were going to be hectic or difficult.

And the very odd thing is that nothing factual has actually changed in my life at all. I haven't fallen in love or won the lottery – I just feel as if I have! I do hope you enjoy reading this book, and that you find it easy to use the formulas. Because once you have got your life into the right balance, you are going to sail ahead.

Balance Benefits:
- ✓ More physical energy
- ✓ Ability to deal with problems
- ✓ More personal confidence
- ✓ More enjoyment of everyday life
- ✓ Rediscovering how to have fun

Five:Two
The Golden Balance

Once you start managing your life the Five:Two way, it's amazing to discover that it is all around us. For many, the first time we meet Five:Two is in the dieting principle, where you eat all you want for five days each week and then fast for the other two days. You'll soon discover that it extends far beyond diet, and can provide solutions to so many of our day-to-day worries.

For your health

There's much more to the principle than only how we eat. It's there in the way most of us divide our week up into five days work and two days rest. Our health also seems to fall naturally into this pattern. Guidelines recommend two hours of exercise every five days. Health experts want us to balance drinking wine or spirits by having five small glasses of water or a soft drink for every two small glasses of alcohol.

For your well-being

We know it works for physical health and fitness, and now it's even beginning to look as if Five:Two is the mind's instinctive way of healing itself. Studies are researching what happens when people go through terrible life events like war, accidents and abuse. People who have experienced these often suffer from post-traumatic stress syndrome (PTSS), where they are unable to move on, leading to depression and other illnesses. By comparing those who do cope successfully with those who don't, psychologists have discovered that if we allow our mind to keep revisiting events little by little, in a Five:Two pattern, we can reduce the risk of PTSS.

For family and relationships

When it comes to our family life, counsellors are finding that just two periods of quality time together can mend the problems that arise over the five days of the school or working week. Couples forced into long-distance relationships say the same thing – just two long phone calls or e-chats every five days makes all the difference.

To beat the years

The good news is that Five:Two works all through your life – and even better as you get older. All you need to do is use two of the Beat the Years formulas every five days and you can improve a host of age-related problems including bone-thinning (osteoporosis); movement and stiffness; mental slowness; loneliness. You can even combat those wrinkles.

The Golden Ratio

The idea of having balance and proportion in life has been believed for a long time. Most of the world's religions understand that you need to have at least one or two days every week to rest, relax and pray or meditate. The science was added around the time of Leonardo da Vinci, when the Golden Ratio was discovered. Originally used in art and architecture, the idea was that there was a natural proportion for all things, and this would be pleasing and harmonious. Now this book takes that concept into our daily lives, so we can all find a balance that works for us as individuals.

Chunking

Luckily it doesn't take a genius like da Vinci to understand the idea of putting balance into life. When scientists and researchers talk about ratios and proportions, there's quite a straightforward way of putting it – Chunking. Our ratio is really simple: five Chunks on one side, balanced with two Chunks on the other. It's as easy as that. When I first started researching this book I was chatting about Chunking to my old friend Steph (we'll meet her later), and she said, 'Well, you've always chunked your life!' She's right, and I think lots of us do it instinctively, but in a rather random way. With this book we're going to learn how to use Chunking to take control of troublesome areas of our life.

So what is a Chunk? The short answer is: a Chunk is whatever you want it to be.

Here is a Chunk:

Think of a Chunk as an empty box. You can put whatever you want into that box, and that becomes your Chunk. Here are some examples of Chunks:

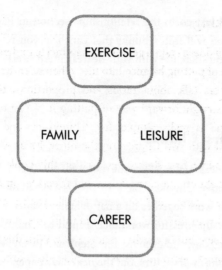

So basically a Chunk is an element of your life that needs balancing. For every five Chunks, you will have two balancing Chunks. This book will show you what balancing Chunks you can use, for whatever you want to improve. Just look through Part Two to see the different sections, which deal with the main topics that we sometimes need help with.

How to use Chunks

Perhaps you need to get healthier and fitter? We can use Chunks of exercise to balance the Chunks where you are sitting at your desk, or like me, at a computer screen. Or maybe your relationships are going through a rocky patch? Just go to the relationships section in Part Two and you will find Chunks that can help you rebalance how you share life with your nearest and dearest.

My first Chunks

Steph was right when she pointed out that I am an instinctive Chunker. Back in the day, when she and I used to work together on a national newspaper, we were in a really stressful workplace. I used to Chunk up my working day, and even my life. Steph and I were working very long hours getting out the next day's paper. Looking back I can see that I had Chunks of five work and two relaxation. My work Chunks were an hour long, and my rest Chunks were ten minutes long. I would have loved the rest Chunks to be longer, but with the pressure of deadlines it wasn't possible. Still, for every five work Chunks, I had two rest Chunks, and it helped.

I tended to Chunk up working life separately from the rest of my life, which I felt suited me at the time. So initially I would have five day-long Chunks of work, followed by two day-long Chunks of home life, but as I got promoted, I needed to change this Chunking strategy. I was either working or on-call pretty much every day – yes, even including Christmas Day. The only day a national newspaper shuts is Christmas Eve, because that's the only day of the year there won't be a paper on the streets the next day.

If I had known about the principle then, I could have worked out a Chunking strategy to help me balance my life. My friend Steph's solution was to blend the two together. Now we look back on it, we can see that she was using small-size Chunks, so every day had its own balance of work and home life.

Are you a Chunker?

Do you instinctively Chunk? Do you think about doing two things for yourself for every five things you do for other people? Lots of us do that. We spend most of our time rushing round acting as chauffeurs to our children; private secretaries to our partners; agony aunts to our family and friends; unpaid charity workers for the local community – but every once in a while we call a halt and do something for ourselves. At least we should do. And that's where this book comes in. If you are finding it hard to Chunk or if you think you might be Chunking already, this book can show you how to achieve more with your Chunking.

What might you Chunk?

If you are already a bit of a Chunker you can probably spot what areas of your life you Chunk. Maybe like me, you tend to Chunk work up. Or perhaps you've already been on the Five:Two diet (also known as the Fast Diet) and learned how to Chunk days of normal eating with periods of fasting. But have you thought that Chunking could help you cut down on alcohol? Perhaps you are beginning to feel age catching up with you? Chunking up the way you manage the ageing process can help you wind back the years.

What size is a Chunk?

The Chunk box can be as big or as little as it needs to be, as long as each five Chunks have two balancing Chunks. Sometimes Chunks might contain a really major life event, like having a baby. Other Chunks might be just about small things, like trying to cut down on coffee. At the moment, I'm really excited about writing this book, so I'm giving it five Chunks. But I'm also determined to run a full marathon for charity, so I'm going to balance my five writing Chunks with two Chunks of running, which will be an ideal off-set for sitting at the computer. In Part Two you will see how flexible the Chunks are, so that many of the things in your life can be coped with more easily by applying a bit of Chunking.

Time Chunks

A lot of people like to organize their Chunks by time. A Chunk might be anything from ten minutes to an hour, or even a week or a month. The length of time depends on what it is you are Chunking. So with the Five:Two diet, the Chunks are each a day long – five days normal eating, two days fasting. But a Chunk doesn't have to be a day. It could be a week or a month. Some people use Chunking to slow down a hectic partying lifestyle. For five weeks they party as normal, then the next two weeks they don't drink or party, which gives their body a chance to rest and detox.

Action Chunks

Time isn't always the right way to divide up your Chunks. Sometimes your goal is to do with life events or long-term ambitions. With these things, time isn't necessarily the major issue. It's more a question of what you are actually doing. Someone who is fed up with their current job might have lots of action Chunks. So for every five things they do at work, they will have two action Chunks aimed at improving their work situation.

Here are some examples of Action Chunks:

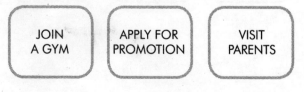

Chunking on your own

Once you've got the habit of Chunking, you won't need this book at all. As soon as you feel things are getting out of hand, or your life is out of balance, you can do some Chunking. Maybe you feel harassed because your children are making too many demands on you? Or perhaps you know you are spending too much time on Facebook and you really need to get out more. Well, just spare a moment to Chunk it.

Here are some empty Chunk boxes for you to fill in to suit yourself:

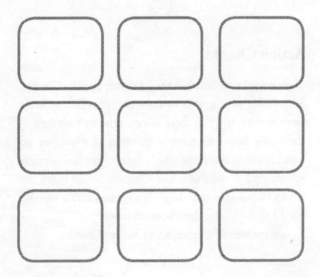

Chunking together

To get started though, it's best to choose one of the plans in Part Two to help you get going and you might find more than one plan is relevant. Even if you are desperate to do more than one, I suggest doing one after the other rather than all at once.

Five:Two can make some very dramatic and long-lasting changes to the way you live, so it's best to give yourself time to adapt. And remember, those around you may also need a little time to adjust to the new you.

Which **Five:Two** Plan for You?

Time to start thinking about using the Five:Two methods in your life. What areas do you think will help you most? Here are the areas this book covers:

1. **Fitness**   Does it feel like you're just too busy to fit fitness in? You know you should do it, but when? This book will show you techniques to get the maximum out of your time, from Fartlek to Tabata to HIIT training, to stretching and breathing techniques. Just two days a week of this fitness regime will get you in the shape you want to be. The good news is that these methods have been used by elite athletes for years.

2. **Work/Life Balance**   We all know there's meant to be one, but sometimes getting a work/life balance seems impossible. Here are the techniques for putting work back in its place, and reclaiming your weekend. This book shows you how to approach your boss for work-at-home time, whether to consider job-share, and could you do better by going self-employed?

3. **Relationships**   Working away from home? Long-distance love? Or just a tired old routine? Using

the methods described in this book can re-enliven relationships and help you through those difficult patches.

4. **Beat the Years** Age seems to be catching up quicker than ever, but did you know that Oxford University medical researchers are suggesting new ways of keeping young? Top-up your full spectrum light for just two days a week and your vitamin D levels will soon be high enough to help fight age-related fatigue. Perform weight training just two hours a week and you can help prevent the onset of osteoporosis. The body's natural rhythms work on a Five:Two cycle, so adjusting your beauty regime to fit will have successful results. Even if you're not getting your beauty sleep you can still use the cycle to get the rest and refreshment you need. And you can schedule beauty treatments to get the best results.

5. **Partying and Social Media** Is the social whirl getting too much? Have those drinks on a Friday night turned into a seven-night marathon? Clinical research has shown how the body can be helped into rapid, healthy recovery by using Five:Two. This is a regime that will help you eliminate the bad effects of too much partying, and help you manage your social drinking and behaviour in the future. Are you addicted to your mobile? Do you Tweet more than is good for you? Or are you fanatical about Facebook? You will be shown a simple technique for breaking addictions to social media and television, without having to give up the fun completely.

6. **Parenting**   It's vital for our children to have quality time with us, but sometimes there just doesn't seem to be the time for it. Here you will be given great schedules for using two minutes, two hours and two days a week to improve the quality of your relationship with your children and give them all the help and love they need.

7. **Well-Being**   You're not depressed exactly, but things have been better. Or maybe you are finding it hard to get over a divorce or a recent death of a loved one. Or there might be issues in your past that you need to revisit. Thanks to the latest psychological research, Five:Two has plenty of solutions to offer.

Choosing your first plan

One of my family and friends who will be testing Five:Two is Mary, who wants to do all the plans at once! Another tester, Stew, is convinced that the Fitness plan is the only one for him. Steph wants to go for the Beat the Years plan. I know all three of them really well, and I actually think Steph might be better off looking at the Work/Life Balance plan first. I do agree with Stew that if Fitness is the big thing for him right now, then he should get stuck into it. But Mary needs to try to think a bit more about what is making her so desperate to change all areas of her life. I wonder if she should start off with the Well-Being plan?

It's not necessarily as easy as it seems to choose the right plan to start with. Chatting with Mary she said: 'Well, if I have to choose just one, it would have to be Relationships. I'm always having huge rows with my husband these days.'

I wondered why Mary and her husband are having rows now, when I can remember they always used to have a great marriage, with lots of shared jokes. Might there be something else wrong, at a deeper level, that's causing Mary to pick fights with her husband? Might she be unhappy about something else, and she's just taking it out by rowing? In other words, might the relationship issue be just a symptom of a more important problem? It can be very hard to tell.

Life is like a pizza

So how do you choose? The good news is that if you can choose a pizza topping, you can choose the right plan.

Here are seven 'life pizzas' for you to choose from; each one has different toppings. Look at all the different 'life pizzas' and see which one has the most toppings that you want to follow up. So if the pizza that speaks to you has toppings like: 'feeling flabby', 'want to be fitter' and 'I'm out of shape', you won't be surprised to discover that's the Fitness pizza.

The Life Pizza Menu

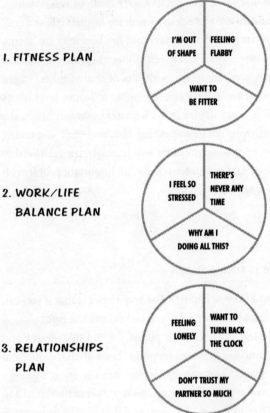

I. FITNESS PLAN

I'M OUT OF SHAPE

FEELING FLABBY

WANT TO BE FITTER

2. WORK/LIFE BALANCE PLAN

I FEEL SO STRESSED

THERE'S NEVER ANY TIME

WHY AM I DOING ALL THIS?

3. RELATIONSHIPS PLAN

FEELING LONELY

WANT TO TURN BACK THE CLOCK

DON'T TRUST MY PARTNER SO MUCH

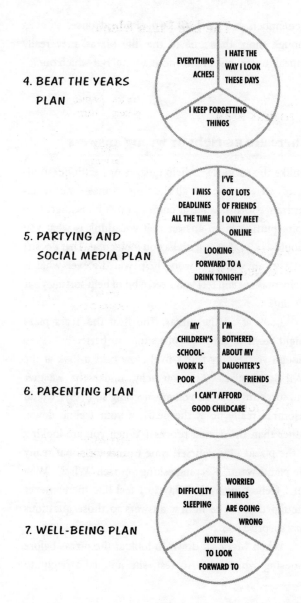

4. BEAT THE YEARS PLAN

EVERYTHING ACHES!
I HATE THE WAY I LOOK THESE DAYS
I KEEP FORGETTING THINGS

5. PARTYING AND SOCIAL MEDIA PLAN

I MISS DEADLINES ALL THE TIME
I'VE GOT LOTS OF FRIENDS I ONLY MEET ONLINE
LOOKING FORWARD TO A DRINK TONIGHT

6. PARENTING PLAN

MY CHILDREN'S SCHOOLWORK IS POOR
I'M BOTHERED ABOUT MY DAUGHTER'S FRIENDS
I CAN'T AFFORD GOOD CHILDCARE

7. WELL-BEING PLAN

DIFFICULTY SLEEPING
WORRIED THINGS ARE GOING WRONG
NOTHING TO LOOK FORWARD TO

Remember, you can't eat two pizzas at once, so even though more than one of the 'life pizzas' may really appeal to you, just order one at a time. But which one?

There are no right or wrong answers

Unlike the various self-help quizzes or health questionnaires we come across all the time in magazines or on insurance forms, when it comes to this book there's no point putting in an answer that you think is what you should say, or that will make you look good. That doesn't get you anywhere. It won't help you discover what is really making you feel you need a bit of help sorting your life out.

Look at all the pizzas. The Beat the Years pizza might seem to sum up your situation perfectly – even though you're only thirty-five! Now have a look at the Well-Being pizza. Are you achy, under the weather and forgetful because you are sleeping so badly? Could insomnia really be at the heart of your feeling down, rather than the ageing process? When you are looking at the pizzas give yourself time to think: 'Is that really the plan I want?' Keeping asking yourself 'Why?': 'Why am I feeling lonely?'; 'Why do I feel like there's never enough time?' The honest answers to those questions may surprise you.

When Mary sat down to look at the pizzas before choosing which plan to test, she jumped straight to the pizza that said: 'I feel so stressed'; 'There's never any time'; 'Why am I doing all this?' Mary said: 'That's me in a nutshell, you must have been thinking of me when you wrote it.' I wasn't. But I was thinking of Mary when I created the Well-Being pizza: 'I have difficulty sleeping; I'm worried things are going wrong'; 'I've nothing to look forward to'. It took a lot of persuading to get Mary to look at that plan first – we'll find out more about what she did and how she got on later.

See the whole picture

If it helps, feel free to read through the whole book before you get started on your own personal plan. The idea of the Five:Two ratio is really down to common sense, and learning how to develop a feeling of balance and proportion in your life.

The earliest civilizations agreed with the idea that all human beings benefited from having balance in life, and 2,000 years ago, the Romans coined the phrase 'A sound mind in a healthy body' to sum it up. That phrase is misused a lot these days to push people down to the gym. Really it means that the things we do with our minds should be positive ('sound'), and that our minds should be supported by a balancing framework of the other things in our lives. Those are usually physical, but they aren't just exercise. They could be relaxation, leisure pursuits, social interaction.

Find the right balance for all these aspects of who you are, and you will discover your whole life opening out. Things that seemed impossible will suddenly become quite easy. Think of a big see-saw with a sack of potatoes on one end and a biscuit on the other. While all those heavy potatoes are weighing down the bottom end, you are never going to be able to move that top end down so you can reach the biscuit (it's smothered in chocolate, by the way). But start moving some of those potatoes, and soon the see-saw will be in balance, and the biscuit will be within reach.

Meet the Testers

Time flies when you're having fun, and I'm amazed to realize that I have been following research into health and lifestyle for more than twenty-five years. It all started when I was a journalist on a national newspaper, and one of my jobs was to research and write the latest diets for readers, which we would serialize regularly in the newspaper. Ten years later my books on slimming and lifestyle were being published, and since then I've always been involved with the latest research findings.

The good news is that as scientists and medical experts discover more about how to stay healthy and happy into old age, the Five:Two ratio is popping up again and again. We now understand why it is a really effective way for people to lose weight and keep it off. Sports scientists are also finding the evidence to back up what elite athletes have known for years – that fitness improves much better if high activity is balanced with recovery periods. The science of gerontology, research into ageing, is pointing the same way, and coming up with results that show people can stay active and healthy into old age when they incorporate Five:Two methods to maintain their lifestyles. For this book, though, I wanted to conduct my own research to make sure that 'the golden balance' really can work across our daily lives. Does it have answers to the broad spectrum of challenges we all come up with from time to time?

I decided to carry out my own experiment. So I recruited family and friends to test the ideas in this book. While it was being researched and written, they have been acting as 'test pilots' to see how well the recipes work in their lives. They have been reporting back to me all the way, over a coffee or at a family get-together – but more often with constant texts and emails, sometimes delighted, sometimes doubtful, and occasionally downright flabbergasted!

Every experiment has to have what's called a 'control group'. The control group just continues life as normal, so that their results can be compared with those who have been taking part in the experiment. Appropriately, there are five testers, whom I've called the 'test pilots' and two in the control group – I suppose that makes them the 'air controllers'. Their experiences and comments will be included throughout the book, so let's meet them . . .

The test pilots

Stew

In his younger days, Stew, thirty-six, was a semi-pro athlete in the worlds of body building and martial arts. Now he's self-employed and building his own business rather than his body. Like a lot of former sportsmen, he's never really had to think about a healthy lifestyle before, and it's come as a big surprise to him that his body is beginning to let him down. Stew wants to get back in shape again but doesn't know if he can fit it in with working twenty-four/seven on the business. So he will be particularly interested in the exercise section of the book. I suspect we are going to be hearing a lot from him about the sweaty bits.

Mary

In her mid-sixties, Mary is now retired from full-time work but continues to work part-time for the government carrying out civil service department reviews. She also has a few private and charitable board directorships. Her three sons are all more or less at home in between travelling, university and difficulties in today's job market. And her retired husband makes four men on the scene to be looked after – no wonder Mary feels harassed and hectic. She wants to apply Five:Two in her work/life balance, relationships, anti-ageing . . . In fact, she says: 'More or less everything, except parenting – I've done more than enough of that.'

Mark

Mark is the youngest of the test pilots. He's still at university and has recently got a bit worried about his partying. 'It never occurred to me that it could be getting over the top, but I had a work placement this summer, and if I'm really truthful, it was harsh.' Mark turned up late a few times, and when his boss explained how much importance he placed on the problem, Mark had to take it seriously. But he found it much harder than he had expected to adjust his lifestyle to the demands of a working environment. He's now seriously questioning whether he is spending too much time gaming, on social media, and partying. Those are the sections of this book he knows he needs to test.

Steph

Steph and her husband are a two-career couple with three young children, and she says: 'I don't know if things are going well, I haven't had time to check.' She feels almost every section of the book is relevant: parenting, relationships and work/life balance – 'The lot!' Secretly though, Steph confessed to me that she is also particularly interested in the anti-ageing section, as she approaches the big 4-0 birthday.

Me

The final test pilot is me. At present I'm obviously very busy researching and writing this book, but I do have my hands full on a number of other fronts. I'm about to run a 26.2 mile marathon in aid of charity, and I'm fairly involved in local community organizations and charity work, and I'm also training a spaniel puppy, and looking after two horses, and also not forgetting the day job, journalism, also . . . also . . . With the marathon coming up, I'm particularly interested in the exercise recipes. Like Steph, I'm keen to see how the anti-ageing methods work – but in my case, at fifty-five, the anti-ageing is considerably more urgent than for a babe like Steph.

The air controllers

Rob

Rob really wanted to be one of the test pilots but I wouldn't let him – somebody has to be in the control group. Rob's recently divorced and he's worried he will lose touch with his children as he has to work abroad a lot. I think if I had let him, Rob would have wanted to follow the parenting and the relationships sections. Although he's in reasonably good shape, with so much travelling he does find it hard to fit exercise in. After chatting about his role, Rob and I have agreed that although he's not yet going to use this programme, he will keep in touch with all of us test pilots and see how things develop. If he still wants to join later on, we've decided he can, as long as it doesn't impact on the experiment.

Melanie

Melanie is the ideal air controller because she really doesn't agree with the idea of the book at all. I asked her to be a control because I think she has the perfect life, which means that it will be a really good test of this principle if we can impress her. Melanie, twenty-eight, is single and works in London. She goes to the gym most mornings before work and usually goes out with her friends for a quick drink after work. She often works overtime from home at weekends but then on other weekends she might go to a festival with friends. Mel says she visits her parents every month (I'm not so sure it's that regular). When it comes to some of the recipes, she doesn't think two hours a week is anything like enough exercise. And she doesn't see any reason to introduce two no-party days into her week since she's already in good shape. She's agreed that she will let me know if her life is continuing to be as enviable as ever while the rest of us get stuck into Five:Two.

Good luck everyone, here we go!

Setting Your
Five:Two Goals

Knowing what you want to achieve is every bit as important as finding out how to achieve it. Yet surprisingly few of us really do know exactly what we want out of life. One of our test pilots, Mary, is always saying to me, 'Oh, one day I'm going to move to France.' I'm just as bad – my catchphrase is: 'I'm sure I've got a novel in me.' And a friend's husband who works in the City usually comes out with: 'I've always thought I could run a bar' towards the end of our second bottle of wine.

But those aren't proper life-changing goals. They are just our way of expressing that we don't think we've got a good balance in our lives. And Five:Two is all about putting the balance into your life. This goal-setting plan will help you to identify the particular parts of your life that Five:Two is going to help. As you get used to the technique, you'll find you can bring your whole life into balance, and that's when it gets exciting. You're going to turn vague 'I wish' and 'I might' into 'I will' and 'I can'. To do that, you first need to set your goals, and this section shows you how. Read through it, then sit down on your own somewhere quiet and have a think. When you're ready, you can write down your goal at the end of this section.

First of all, let's discover the **PASTA** method to define for yourself a goal that is:

P	positive
A	achievable
S	sensible
T	tickable
A	actual

Positive

Use only positive phrases when setting your goal: 'I will do'; 'I can do'; 'I like'; 'I want to'.

Beware of negative terms: 'I am not going to spend so much time watching TV,' because psychologists have discovered your subconscious mind doesn't hear the 'not', so responds as though you were telling yourself to 'spend much time watching TV'. This is a big problem when you want to give something up, like smoking or overeating, because you have to phrase that goal in positive terms. So: 'I want to eat healthily now' not: 'I'm not eating junk foods any more.'

Make sure you are aiming at a positive outcome: 'I will try for this promotion because I know I can bring something to the job.' Not: 'I'm going for this promotion to spite Sarah because she really wants that job.'

Achievable

Your goals must be possible for you personally to achieve in the real world. Aiming at something that you know in your heart of hearts you can't ever achieve will turn you off the whole programme. Just because a celebrity has swum the River Thames doesn't mean that is achievable for you.

Beware of setting impossible goals and then beating yourself up for failing to achieve them. Research has shown that it's a way for people to find an excuse for not trying. A dieter will say: 'My goal weight is nine stone,' but if she was never nine stone even as a teenager, we all know this isn't achievable. Instead the goal should be: 'I want to lose a stone over the next six months.'

Test pilot Steph needs to have a think about her anti-ageing goal and realize that she can never actually set the clock back – no matter how hard she tries, that big 4-0 is going to come round. So she's going to work on an anti-ageing goal that is achievable, and she'll be reporting back on that later.

Setting achievable goals won't restrict you. You can use them as stepping stones towards a bigger goal. The more achievable your goal, the more likely it is that you will really try to achieve it, and succeed.

Sensible

A sensible goal is relevant to your life, your needs, your talents and your abilities. By setting yourself sensible goals you can really enhance your life and feel better about yourself. But if your goal is random, and doesn't really mean anything to you, even achieving it may not be as helpful as you had hoped.

When he heard I was training for a marathon, a friend of mine told me his goal was to run in the London Marathon next spring. Not only had he never run before, but he hadn't discovered that just getting an entry to the London Marathon is an achievement in itself. So it really wasn't a sensible goal for him, and sure enough, he never got started. When you begin your fitness plan, having the goal of winning the Tour de France or getting an Olympic medal really isn't sensible – unless you happen to be Bradley Wiggins or Mo Farah.

Tickable

For a goal to work for you, there must be a moment when you know you have actually achieved it. So there has to be a box for you to tick. This means you should be careful to define exactly what your goal is. It's no good having a goal that says: 'I want to be thinner.' How much thinner? Thinner than you were yesterday? Or thinner than you will be tomorrow – if you are planning to eat a Chinese takeaway tonight, you already are thinner than you will be tomorrow. Instead your goal should be: 'I want to get my hip measurement down to thirty-six inches.' On the glorious morning when the tape actually does read thirty-six inches, you know you can tick that box. You have achieved your goal.

When test pilot Stew got started, he said his goal was: 'To get back to the shape I used to be in.' But the shape Stew used to be in was winning martial arts competitions, so that would have to be the tick box. Stew emailed me: 'Having to rethink that, no way I'm doing another martial arts comp.' So now he's trying to work out a tickable goal that will achieve his aim of getting in better shape – I wonder what he'll come up with?

Actual

Being vague is probably one of the biggest obstacles to achieving a happy, balanced life. It's something we are all guilty of. How often have you heard people say: 'Oh, one day I'm going to move to Europe,' or 'I'd love to run a country hotel'? These aren't statements of intent at all, they are just our way of saying we are not really happy with our lives just at the moment.

Instead take a moment to think about how you feel, read through this section carefully, and then try to plan an actual goal. So, instead of saying how much you'd love to have a guest house in the countryside, set yourself the actual goal of researching what it takes to run one. Your goal then would be: 'Six months from now I will know what the costings would be; I will have talked to people who do it; I will have a thorough understanding of what is involved and know if I still want to consider it.' Then your next goal might be: 'Five years from now I will be running a little hotel in the countryside.'

Test pilot Stew sets his goal

When we sat down to do Stew's goals, he told me: 'I was in great shape when I was in my twenties, I want to be like that again.' Alarm bells sounded – this was going to fail the PASTA test. First of all I asked Stew if he thought his goal was Positive? 'Sure, what could be more positive than aiming to be in great shape, like I was in my twenties?' But actually, isn't it rather negative to aim to go back to where you were ten years ago? You're a big boy now, Stew, with your own business to run. Wouldn't it be more positive to accept who you are now and aim to be in the best shape a busy grown-up businessman can be?

'Yeah, and the other thing I'm worried about is that I'm physically older now,' confessed Stew. 'It was tough enough back then; heaven knows what it's going to be like now.' So Stew's initial goal also fails the Achievable test.

Most blokes and plenty of women will agree that you just can't do what you used to be able to do in your twenties, whether it's winning your local tennis tournament or partying all night.

And is it Sensible? As a young man, Stew's sports were body building and martial arts. Is that the kind of impression he wants to give when approaching clients in his new computer software business? 'Well, it depends,' concedes Stew. 'All right, then, not really.'

So, not Positive or Achievable or Sensible. What about Tickable? In other words, is there a box that Stew will be able to tick on a particular day that says: Yes, I have achieved that goal? 'Obviously not,' says Stew, 'because it's just a kind of all-round fitness thing really.' And, to cap it all, there's no way a vague statement like 'all-round fitness' would tick the Actual box.

We arrived at a goal that Stew liked and that fitted PASTA really well. He decided that his goal was to take part in a triathlon competition (swim, bike, run) being held in his area in the spring. Here's how his Triathlon goal fitted PASTA:

Stew's
PASTA Goal-Setting Planner

	Goal	To compete in a triathlon next spring	
P	**positive**	*There will be all-round health benefits without pushing Stew too hard*	✓
A	**achievable**	*Lots of people Stew's age enjoy triathlons as a hobby, and there's no requirement to win!*	✓
S	**sensible**	*Stew already swims with his son once a week and occasionally cycles to his office, so there's a sensible opportunity for him to step this up enough to do a triathlon in a few months*	✓
T	**tickable**	*The day of the triathlon will come in six months, and Stew either competes and ticks the box, or not*	✓
A	**actual**	*Rather than a vague wish, the triathlon is an actual event*	✓

My own PASTA goal

I've been teasing Stew about how vague his original idea of a goal was, but I have to admit that even though I've been using the PASTA formula for years, my own current wishes and hopes were just as far from being a proper PASTA goal as Stew's. Time to confess! I've been a freelance author and journalist for quite a few years now, but like a lot of self-employed people, my business took quite a hit when the recession started. So I want to get my work back to where it was before then. But that's just as imprecise as Stew's original goal so I had to do some thinking, and here's how my PASTA goal-setting planner looks:

Janet's PASTA Goal-Setting Planner

	Goal	To write Five:Two for a new you	
P	positive	*This will help lots of readers to improve the balance in their lives, as well as boosting my work*	✓
A	achievable	*I've written lots of books already, so I know I can do this*	✓
S	sensible	*My editor likes the concept of the book so far, so it's not just me wanting to do it*	✓
T	tickable	*When the book is published, I can tick that I have done it*	✓
A	actual	*There will be a book for everyone to read at the end of the day*	✓

Now over to you – here's your goal chart

This is the fun bit – you get to set your own goal. If you are like me and have lots of different goals, start by just setting one goal, the most important one. So have a think about which of the various life plans seems most relevant to you at the moment, and set your goal in that area first.

Don't worry if your goal is short-term, and might only take a month or so to achieve. Once you have achieved it, just tick the box and then move on to setting your next goal. If you have lots of different goals in mind, photocopy the goal-setting planner before you fill it in, so you can use it again next time. But remember – it's best to do just one goal at a time.

Your PASTA Goal-Setting Planner

	Goal		
P	**positive**		
A	**achievable**		
S	**sensible**		
T	**tickable**		
A	**actual**		

PART TWO
The **Five:Two** Plans

The **Five:Two**
Fitness Plan

The most exciting thing about this book is that it makes such big differences so quickly. Like all good solutions, it gives you the feeling of being completely natural and obvious – that 'Why on earth haven't I always done this?' moment. And of course, everyone can do it. The Fitness Plan introduces exercise into your life in a balanced way. It combines fitness days with rest days, and is achievable for most people.

Expert guidelines

When official health experts first began to issue fitness guidelines, they called for forty minutes of aerobic exercise at least three times a week. We, the general public, didn't show a lot of enthusiasm for that – to put it mildly.

The health experts soon realized that people need goals that are achievable – something that this book understands very well. People were put off by the impossible official fitness targets, so didn't bother at all. Meanwhile, researchers in the rapidly growing science of fitness began to discover that there are many different ways of achieving improved fitness. Originally, regular long sessions of moderate-intensity exercise – like jogging or swimming – were thought to be the only way to get fit. Then sports scientists discovered that people who did short, sharp bursts of intense, hard exercise, also reached the peaks of fitness.

Enjoy yourself

So it doesn't have to be just running. Sports science is now showing that all sorts of different activities, from team sports, to martial arts, to weight training, to aerobic classes – even dancing – all improve our fitness, health and well-being. It's a little bit like the story of the tortoise and the hare, except that with fitness, both the tortoise and the hare can win. So go on, enjoy yourself. There's bound to be the right activity out there for you.

Fitness Chunks

Reacting to the lack of enthusiasm shown by the public for those tough exercise guidelines, health experts have now revised their thinking with a much more flexible Five:Two style of approach. As long as we put in our two hours a week of exercise, experts now say we can divide it up however suits us.

On the Fitness Plan we are going to use Chunking to break up our exercise routines into bite-size Chunks that are easy to achieve and better for all-round health and well-being. The good news is that Five:Two methods have been used by elite athletes for years. This book shows you the training techniques to get the maximum out of your time, including Fartlek, Tabata and HIIT. When he read that, test pilot Stew texted me: 'Hang on I'm not farting around'. Calm down, Stew! Check out the training technique boxes and you can see that Fartlek is the name for a method of training. It comes from Swedish and means 'speed play', allowing you to play with different speeds during your exercise. The classic Fartlek combination is five periods of less intense work, followed by two hard, and then back to five slower to recover.

Fartlek

Continuous interval training for runners and cyclists, session lasts about forty-five minutes varying between light, moderate and hard

---

Five slow: Two fast

While researching and writing this book I have been training to run a 26.2 mile full marathon in aid of a local charity. My mid-training goal was to run the Bristol Half Marathon of thirteen miles. Come the day, of course, I hadn't really done enough training, but I was still determined to get round. By about the seventh mile, things were really not going well, and many negative thoughts about my age and my work were entering my mind. Traffic cones were placed along the road about every 100 metres, so I decided I would run steadily past five of them, then put on a little spurt of speed for the next two.

It worked really well and I was soon in a good rhythm. But at around mile eleven, I had to do it again – this time a lot slower. I did five cones running and then two walking. Embarrassing, I know . . . A banana, a Batman, and a load of soldiers in full combat gear trudged past me, but Five:Two got me home.

Five:Two fitness works for everyone

You don't have to be running a marathon to use the techniques you will learn in the fitness plan. Just two days a week of *Five:Two For a New You* fitness training will soon get you in the shape you want to be. There are lots of different ways to Chunk up your fitness. Many health professionals swear by:

* Two days of one hour a day
* Five days of twenty minutes a day (three or four days is also OK)
* Two very hard minutes every session

Two hours, twenty minutes, two minutes

Following this system is very flexible. It works well for most people, and it still fits in with what the health and fitness experts recommend. It means that you only have to put in an hour-long exercise session on two days a week. Choose these training sessions from the fitness formulas below. You might choose to go running for those sessions, or go to the gym, or even have a personal trainer. The other five days a week all you need is just twenty minutes doing something gentle that works with your daily life. A brisk walk or a cycle ride are the usual options, but some people walk up and down the stairs or even skip. As you get fitter and keener, you can select your twenty-minute sessions from the fitness formulas as well.

Every session you do, whether it's an hour or just twenty minutes, should include one two-minute interval where you really are trying very hard and feeling pretty sweaty. By the end of each week you will have achieved a really good all-round level of exercise, at a pace that suits you.

How hard should I try?

I sometimes go running with a friend who is a personal trainer, but not often, because he has the very irritating habit of skipping along backwards in front of me chatting about a movie, while I am toiling sweatily away at maximum effort. Everybody's 'hard' is different. Those who've never exercised before, or are overweight, are going to find stuff hard that other people don't even lose breath over.

How hard exercise feels can also depend on how you feel mentally. If you don't enjoy a particular activity it will feel a lot harder than something you like doing. And if you are in a bad mood or having an off day, exercise that is normally OK suddenly seems almost impossible.

Heart rates

To get a more accurate measure of how hard they are training, athletes and serious exercisers check how fast their heart is beating. This is called heart-rate Beats Per Minute (BPM). Our hearts have a maximum BPM, above which we can't go any harder. For some very fit young athletes the maximum could be as high as 190 BPM or even 200 BPM, but for the rest of us it's lower, depending on our age and fitness. Comparing the heart rate BPM while exercising against the maximum possible BPM gives us a good idea of exactly how hard we are training.

How hard are you working?

Using heart-rate BPM monitoring can be quite complicated, so sports scientists have developed an alternative method that works fine for regular exercise programmes. This is called 'perceived exertion' – in other words, how hard does it feel? They've worked out five levels of exercise from very light to maximum, which match up with the heart-rate BPM zones. Using the heart-rate zone chart below can tell us how hard we are exercising without the need to monitor our heart rate. See table on next page.

Aim for: five twenty-minute sessions a week of very light to moderate (three or four is also OK) or two-hour-long sessions of moderate with two minutes of hard to maximum in every session.

Medical note

Please, please promise me that if you have never exercised before you will see a doctor before you start. Your blood pressure, resting heart rate, blood glucose and cholesterol level all need to be checked to make sure they are normal. Doctors can usually spare the time to do this, and are very keen for us to get our health checked.

If you are already following Five:Two diet methods, be warned that it's not a very good idea to have your two long exercise sessions on the same days as your two fasting days. Some people manage it, but it tends to be those who are already quite fit and near their goal weight.

Heart-Rate Zones

Exertion level	Feels like	Good for	Who can do it?	Heart zone	Heart-rate BPM
Very light	Easy and relaxing	All-round health and well-being	Beginners, recovery from injury or illness	50% (of max) *metabolic*	100–114
Light	Comfortable but aware of breathing	Weight loss, start of fitness plan	Everybody from beginners to endurance	60–70% *fat burner*	114–133
Moderate	Slightly hard, getting warmer, breathing quicker but can still talk	Improves fitness and stamina	Intermediate exercisers and specialist training	70–80% *aerobic*	133–152
Hard	Sweaty, breathing hard, muscles aching, but OK	Takes performance up a notch	Experienced exercisers to improve	80–90% *anaerobic*	152–171
Maximum	Full on, muscles on fire, breathing difficult to control	A new personal best	Fit, experienced exercisers and elite athletes	90–100% *anaerobic*	171–190

Ready to go!

So now we know how much exercise to do, what shall we do? The choice is up to you. You can pick from one of the five exercise formulas below, or you can mix and match. Because of training for the marathon, I do my two long sessions from the Formula for Stamina and Team Sport, which has the running schedules I need. At the moment I'm also doing a couple of my twenty-minute sessions from that formula as well, because I really need to get the miles in. But for a change of scene, once a week I go to the gym for a session from the Formula for Weight Training.

Test pilot Stew has chosen the Formula for Stamina and Team Sport, because he needs to train to run, bike and swim for his triathlon, and these are all stamina sports. You can either stick to one formula or you can cherry-pick your favourite bits. As long as you get your two hours, twenty minutes, two minutes in you will be fine. Research has shown that people succeed much better in a fitness programme if they choose a sport or exercise type that they are naturally suited to and that they enjoy.

Choose your formula

If you have never exercised before, you're just going to have to experiment. Your body type might give you a hint. If you are quite stocky and naturally muscular, weight training or martial arts might suit you. The more light-framed and lean types usually do better at running. Those who have a tendency to body fat often turn out to be good swimmers. They have natural buoyancy and resistance to cold water, and the slightly greater body mass doesn't matter much in the water.

Were you good at sports at school? How about picking up those team sports again? Being in a team sport is an excellent motivator, as it has a good social side and also forces you to get out and do it, so as not to let the rest of the team down. Adventurous types will find outdoor recreations like climbing or orienteering give them the excitement they are looking for.

Cross-training (where exercise is varied across different sports) has something for everyone, and is the choice of sports scientists. By spreading your fitness regime across a variety of different sports and exercise you gain lots of benefits. The risk of injury is reduced, since you are not overstressing any one part of your body. Your all-round health improves because the different sports work on different elements of your physique. There's less risk of boredom. You are often out in the fresh air. And you can even include your favourite hobbies like dancing or horse riding. What's not to like?

The Five:Two Fitness Formulas

The formula for stamina and team sport

Stamina sports include running, cycling, swimming, power walking. Many team sports, like soccer and rugby, are also stamina sports, as they require you to be able to keep going for about thirty to forty-five minutes at moderate level, with some periods of light and some of hard exercise. If you get serious about your stamina sports you will end up being able to keep going for much longer periods, even of four or five hours. These sports are really good for your heart, your lungs and fat burning.

If you are new to exercising, or coming back after a long break, do not expect to be able to do thirty minutes at moderate level to start with. You will need to build up to it.

Five Chunks of very light, or light exercise – as much as you can comfortably manage – are how you start.

* **Joggers** can use five lamp posts, or five telegraph poles (anything that is about 100 metres apart)
* **Cyclists** should be able to go quite happily for five minutes
* **Swimmers** should do about five metres (one fifth of a length of a normal twenty-five-metre pool) using their most comfortable stroke – even if it's on your back or doggy paddle

Two Chunks of light or moderate exercise – not so comfortable – are what you do next.

* **Joggers** should run rather than jog or walk for the next two lamp posts
* **Cyclists** should pedal harder for the next two minutes
* **Swimmers** should use their fastest stroke and try hard for two metres

Even if you are fairly unfit, you should be able to keep this up for an hour. You might have to make your five Chunks very slow and your two Chunks only a little bit harder. The ratio of Five:Two means that you are getting plenty of time for your body to recover between each period of slightly increased effort. If you do this two hours a week, you will very soon find that you can increase the intensity of your exercise. Where you were doing five Chunks at very light exercise, those five Chunks might now be at light or moderate.

When you feel ready, flip your Chunks over. Now your Chunks of two become your rest Chunks, and your Chunks of five become your effort Chunks.

The final stage is to increase the length of your effort Chunks. Don't rush to do this, let it happen naturally. And remember that no matter how long the effort Chunks, they should still be matched by rest Chunks in the balance of five effort and two rest Chunks.

Runners may soon find that they have run fairly hard for five lamp posts yet still don't need a rest. Their new effort Chunk might then be a mile. Pretty soon it will be five miles, and then it's next stop a marathon!

Cyclists are helped by a miracle of engineering – the bicycle – so more than anybody they will soon find they are able to go long distances without needing to rest. A Chunk of five kilometres is nothing to an experienced cyclist.

Swimmers usually use a length of the average twenty-five-metre pool as a base for their Chunks. Five lengths of moderate swimming, followed by two lengths of light swimming works well. With swimming it's very important to remain in control of your breathing, so you may not be able to step up your exercise level as quickly. A few proper swimming lessons can help tremendously.

Team sports players can use the same formula to get fit for their sport. Team training sessions are usually once a week, so just make that one of your two hour-long sessions and go with the above formula for the other hour-long session.

Remember to include one two-minute burst of very hard exercise in every session. If things go well you can also try interval training:

> **High Intensity Interval Training (HIIT)**
> Famously used by Peter Coe training his son,
> Seb, now Lord Coe, to Olympic success,
> alternates short periods of hard with shorter
> rest periods for up to thirty-minute sessions

The formula for weight training

Weight training is right back in fashion, for some very
sound health reasons. It improves muscular strength all
round – including your heart, which is a muscle. Weight-
bearing exercise greatly reduces the risk of osteoporosis.
A lot of research is also showing that it is as effective
for fat loss as the normally recommended exercises like
running. Many people who are unsuited to running find
that they get a big buzz out of weight training. It has a
good social side with people usually buddying-up in
the gym, and there are lots of different kinds of weight
training. Once shown how, a novice can use machines
which make sure you are doing it properly. There are also
lots of new routines around using light bar weights, kettle
bells and even Indian clubs. Once you get serious, then
you can go on to lifting heavier 'free' weights with a mate
to watch or 'spot' you. Join or guest at a local gym and
there will be trainers available to help you get started.
Here's how a week on the Weight Training Formula will
work:

First one-hour session At the gym. Warm up on exercise bike for ten minutes, building to hard for the last two minutes. Then forty minutes on weight machines supervised (at first) by a gym attendant/trainer. Ten minutes cooling down and stretching.

Second one-hour session At the gym or at home. Using light, free weights – e.g. hand held dumb-bells, perform routines advised by gym. There are also classes available at most gyms using free weights to get you started. Two minutes hard before the end of the session, and ten minutes cooling down and stretching.

Twenty-minute sessions These don't have to be weight training. They can be any form of exercise at any intensity. Recommended is power walking, carrying light hand-held or wrist weights.

The formula for outdoor recreation

This is my favourite formula because it lets you get out and do anything you want. Really, anything – as long as it is something. Here are some of the recreations you could choose (look online for further details of organizations):

Dog walking – if you are experienced, this could even become a bit of a money-spinner

Hill climbing/walking – set yourself a long-term goal to build towards like completing a long-distance path or even climbing Snowdon

Open-water swimming – happens in rivers, lakes and sometimes the sea

Orienteering – using a map to find particular places, and can be done competitively

Adventure Racing – team racing in canoes, on mountain bikes etc., usually over a weekend

Rock climbing – indoor climbing walls are available, and later you can get to grips with the real thing

Horse riding – there are many riding schools and trekking centres round the country

Foraging – a great way to take a walk in the countryside and come back with all sorts of wild food. Do a bit of research on areas and on what you can and can't eat (there's lots of information online) before you set out

Skiing and Boarding – on real snow once in a while, but otherwise on roller skates, skate boards, mountain boards, or even a surf board if you are lucky

- ❖ First hour – do your chosen recreation, or a different one each week
- ❖ Second hour – pick a one-hour session from one of the other formulas
- ❖ Twenty-minute session – any form of light to moderate exercise that works for you

The formula for studio and martial arts class

Studio-based classes include 'spinning' (cycling to fast music); 'Zumba' (dance moves); and 'boxercise' (boxing-style moves but no contact). They are highly motivating, with mounds of music and enthusiasm from the teacher – it can be as much of a high as going out clubbing. Martial arts classes often have a similar feel, with lots of high energy flowing.

The only drawback to this formula is that, at least at first, you will have to pay for classes or join a gym. Classes aren't usually very expensive, and they are well worth it for the personal attention from the teacher. Everybody I've talked to says they also become an important part of your social life. Because you will be getting help from a teacher, all you need to do to get started on this formula is find a class and enrol. Aim to do one hour-long class a week at first, and use your other sessions for more gentle exercise. If you get hooked (and most people do) you can step up to two classes a week, or even do a studio-style session at home.

A lot of studio and martial arts classes already include two-minute bursts of high intensity exercise, and many use the Tabata method:

Tabata ™
Invented by Japanese Professor Izumi Tabata involves 20 seconds *maximum* exercise then 10 seconds *very light exercise* for 4 minutes

---

The formula for cross-training

This is the formula I've followed for almost as long as I can remember, and it involves a whole range of different workout styles in your weekly exercise schedule. I normally do one hour from the Stamina Formula and one hour from the Weight Training Formula. My twenty-minute sessions always include dog walking, and in the summer, open-water swimming. If I have a bit of spare time I often add in an extra hour-long session by doing a studio class or going horse riding.

When I write it down, that seems like an awful lot to me but it never feels like that. Because there's such a variety, and all of it (with the possible exception of running) is so enjoyable it never seems like a chore. And of course, compared with real chores, like ironing or hoovering or the school run, it definitely isn't.

Many successful athletes use these methods all the time, either because their sport demands it or because injury prevents hard training in their chosen discipline. To make it work properly, you need to include both stamina and weight training. The simplest way is:

---

1 × 1 hour : from the stamina formula

1 × 1 hour : from the weight training formula

2 × 20 minutes : from the outdoor recreation formula

1 to 3 × 20 minutes : of light exercise (usually just walking)

The **Five:Two** Work/ Life Balance Plan

This is the plan that will revolutionize your outlook on work and your enjoyment of life. Here you can find out how to evaluate your work/life balance and find its strong and weak points. Then, with the help of the right formula, you can turn everything around. Problems with our work/life balance are the second most commonly reported cause of stress after physical illness. Stress doesn't always come from where you might think. A recent study of the workplace found that executive assistants were often far more stressed than the high-flying executives they assisted. Psychologists found that the heart of the problem for the assistants was that they had very little control over their working day, whereas their bosses had a say in everything.

When it comes to work, Five:Two has solutions for so many of the day-to-day work problems that cause stress. There are formulas for how to deal with difficult bosses, how to balance all the different stress factors in your life, and how to cope with the grind of having a boring job.

So what's the problem?

Most of us like a good moan about work, but have you asked yourself exactly what it is you are moaning about? Is there really a problem? And if there is, what is it exactly? The clearer you are about exactly where your work/life balance is going wrong, the easier it will be to fix it.

If you are lucky enough to love both your job and your two children, the problem that there aren't enough hours in the day becomes a mere matter of organization, by comparison with the huge positives in your life. And if you love your job, it's very likely you will also be good at it, and your bosses will know that, so they will want to keep you happy. So you may find a surprising number of helpful responses when you flag up your issue. Maybe you don't love your job. Even so, give it a chance. Sometimes it isn't your work that is the real cause of your problem, but issues elsewhere in your life that are spilling into work and giving you a negative attitude about everything. To help you get a clearer picture of how you really feel about work and its place in your life, use the Work/Life Balance Checker.

Work/Life Balance Checker

Yes, this is a questionnaire, but there are no right or wrong answers, so I'm afraid you can't cheat and come out perfect. Most of us filling in questionnaires tick the boxes we know we should:

I never consume more than six units of alcohol a week	✓
I always take regular aerobic exercise	✓
I have recently read *War and Peace*	✓

Yeah, right. The trouble is, you may get the best possible score on the questionnaire but you can't fool your body, or yourself. Say what you want to the outside world, but with yourself, where it matters, it's much harder to cheat.

So this questionnaire does exactly what it says in the name. It's a checker. You can use it to explore your own feelings about things, and you may come up with a few surprises. My checker has turned out to be a real eye-opener for me.

Janet's Work/Life Balance Checker

Question	always	sometimes	rarely or never
Do you look forward to Fridays?	✓		
Do you look forward to Mondays?		✓	
Do you work extra at weekends?		✓	
Do you take work home?		✓	
Do you take work on holiday?			✓
Do you put work ahead of family events?			✓
Do you enjoy your work?	✓		
When asked about yourself, do you describe your job first?	✓		
Are you proud of your job?	✓		
Did you always want to work in the type of job you have now?	✓		
Do you have interests and friends outside of work?	✓		
Do you feel you are missing out on life?		✓	
Do you envy people you meet or see on TV?			✓

Like most of us, I'm constantly moaning about work. There's always too much (or occasionally not enough). It's boring. It's stressful. It's preventing me from doing what I really want to do. But in fact, when I look at my ticks, I can see that the truth is very different. Sure, I look forward to Fridays – but sometimes, if I've got a really juicy article to research and write, I look forward to Monday just as much. And goodness me, I'd never thought about it before, but secretly I'm actually quite proud of what I do – no matter what people say about journalists.

An air controller does the checker

Melanie, one of the two 'air controllers', volunteered to do the checker because she loves questionnaires and multiple choice and always aces them. Even when I explained you can't win at this checker, she was confident she would be brilliant.

Melanie's Work/Life Balance Checker

Question	always	sometimes	rarely or never
Do you look forward to Fridays?	✓		
Do you look forward to Mondays?			✓
Do you work extra at weekends?	✓		
Do you take work home?	✓		
Do you take work on holiday?	✓		
Do you put work ahead of family events?	✓		
Do you enjoy your work?		✓	
When asked about yourself, do you describe your job first?	✓		
Are you proud of your job?			✓
Did you always want to work in the type of job you have now?			✓
Do you have interests and friends outside of work?	✓		
Do you feel you are missing out on life?			✓
Do you envy people you meet or see on TV?		✓	

Melanie emailed me: 'Checker came out how I thought it would – big career and good social life.'

I emailed back: 'There aren't really any questions on social life. What about never having wanted to work in the job you are in?'

Melanie replied: 'Well, nobody grows up wanting to be a banker!'

What do you think about Melanie's checker? Do you think she's taking it for granted that her work/life balance is great, when it might not be that wonderful after all?

Over to you

Now it's your turn to fill in the checker. Remember, there are no wrong answers. And what you learn from it may surprise you. It may help you realize that you have got into the habit of assuming that your work/life balance is wrong, or that your job is awful, but in fact you are more content than you think. Or it could point out a real issue that you haven't faced before. Perhaps it might remind you that you've missed a parents' evening or skipped your gran's birthday party. That would certainly be a pointer that your work/life balance has gone wonky.

Your Work/Life Balance Checker

Question	always	sometimes	rarely or never
Do you look forward to Fridays?			
Do you look forward to Mondays?			
Do you work extra at weekends?			
Do you take work home?			
Do you take work on holiday?			
Do you put work ahead of family events?			
Do you enjoy your work?			
When asked about yourself, do you describe your job first?			
Are you proud of your job?			
Did you always want to work in the type of job you have now?			
Do you have interests and friends outside of work?			
Do you feel you are missing out on life?			
Do you envy people you meet or see on TV?			

Thinking about the checker

The results of your checker should help you identify just what it is about your work/life balance that's bothering you. When you tick that you never work at home or at weekends, you may suddenly realize that is actually because your work isn't challenging or interesting enough. Armed with a bit of self-knowledge you can then choose the right formula to get you back where you want to be. If you fill in the checker again in a few months' time, you should see big improvements. Most of us with busy working lives take it for granted that when it comes to work, the less the better. A school leaver or graduate who still hasn't been able to get into the workplace wouldn't agree with that. Neither would someone in their fifties who has recently been made redundant with little chance of getting another job. So having to go to work isn't necessarily the worst thing in the world – not having to might feel a lot worse.

Even so the work/life balance is a difficult circle to square. It's hard to work out where your priorities should be. The Work/Life Formulas will help you with that. Be adaptable, and be prepared to put a bit of positive energy into finding your way forward. You will be making changes to your working life – and changes to yourself as well.

Thinking about your work

Even when everything seems impossible, remember that there's always a solution. If your job really is a disaster area, you can look for other jobs elsewhere or go self-employed. In truth though, there are very few work/life problems that can't be improved with a little creative thinking. You might be able to find a slightly different role within the organization that suits you better; or your job could be adapted to fit around your needs.

The key to making this happen is to communicate. And this doesn't mean just sitting around moaning to anyone who'll listen. Talk sensibly to your HR department, your boss and probably your boss's boss. Prepare what you are going to say beforehand. Be as positive as you possibly can. Start by listing what you do like about your job (make something up if necessary.) and build from there. I was a boss myself for many years, and when people came to me with problems, I hated it. When they turned up with solutions that they had thought out for themselves, it was great – all I had to do was say yes.

The Five:Two Work/Life Formulas

The formula for career success

You know it's out there and you want to go get it. To succeed with high-flying career goals, your work/life balance is going to need to be five work and two other stuff. We sometimes forget that work is part of life, and life is part of work – so you can be enjoying a great work/life balance even at times when you are at the office more or less twenty-four/seven.

When I worked on a national newspaper, I used to get into the office by about 8 a.m., just as the cleaners were leaving, and frequently I didn't finish before midnight or occasionally 2 a.m. Hey, I was young, it was exciting, and I got rapid promotions. But I wish I'd known about Five:Two, because after a few years on daily newspapers, I was shattered. The normal five days' work and two days' weekend isn't going to cut it for career success. You are likely to be working a six- or seven-day week, so you need to know how to rebalance to get the recharge and relaxation you need.

Remember Chunking?

Divide your long working day into Chunks of five hours. You'll probably be doing two or even three five-hour Chunks, definitely not four. Now you can plan your relax and recharge moments into each five-hour chunk. For every five-hour Chunk, have two periods where you relax completely. You can experiment to find out what length rest periods suit you best. Even two minutes will work, as long as you relax completely.

Two minutes Find a quiet place to be alone (yes, in practice it's going to be on the loo). Close your eyes. Focus on breathing slowly and rhythmically, in and out. Feel your forehead and neck muscles relaxing. Imagine you are in your favourite place (probably not the office loo!) and mentally picture your surroundings. Before the two minutes are up remind yourself of something you have accomplished that you feel proud of. Take that with you back into your busy day.

Twenty minutes You have time to get out of the office, so it's really important to do so. Get outside, even if it's raining. Offices are unhealthy places and you need full-spectrum light and fresh air for top brain functioning. Walk round the block focusing on breathing and what you see around you. Let your brain go into neutral. You won't notice it happening, but by the time you get back to your desk, your subconscious brain will have come up with all sorts of solutions and creative ideas.

The formula for coping with a tough boss

Is he a boss or a silverback gorilla? Is she the boss or Cruella De Vil? Whatever, bossy bosses are a huge source of workplace stress. Here's what bossy bosses do wrong:

❖ They make you work too-long hours
❖ They undermine you with negative and nasty remarks
❖ They don't exercise self-control when there's a crisis

❖ They try to make everything your fault when really it's their responsibility
❖ They don't communicate with you
❖ They make you run errands that are not within your job description
❖ They cut you off from other people in the office, whether colleagues or superiors

First of all, let's get one thing clear. A bossy boss is not a successful, effective manager – no matter what he or she may think. Bossy or bullying bosses are usually trying to cover up the fact that they are not on top of their job. Inside they are often feeling very scared and insecure – but it's hard to see this through all the screaming and shouting! It's also very difficult to keep a hold of yourself and your own identity when you are constantly being bullied, so follow these simple steps:

Stay positive For every two negative things your boss says to you, remind yourself of five positive things about yourself. They can be achievements; things people have said about you recently or in the past; or even just that your cat loves you.

Stay connected For every five days make sure you have two days where you meet up with work colleagues outside the office so you can all let off steam. This prevents your boss from isolating you and gives you a safe environment to talk. Never, ever be tempted to text, tweet, blog or mail anything about your boss to anyone else.

Stay rested For every five working days, make sure you have two clear rest days. If your boss is difficult about this, don't argue the toss with him or her. Go to the HR department and explain that you need two days a week as your rest days. Don't make any reference or complaints directly about your boss, just insist on the correct hours for your contract.

Stay on top of things For every five impossible tasks your boss asks you to do, concentrate on the top two tasks that are definitely the most important, and also the most achievable. When your boss flies off the handle, present him or her with the top two things that have been done.

The formula for boosting a boring job

Even the most high-flying career can stall from time to time, and very few of us are lucky enough to go through our working lives without getting stuck in a real grind of a job at some point. My dead-ender came working on a trade magazine edited by an old-school hack who disappeared at bar-opening time each day. There's no need to get stuck in this rut, just get stuck in to making a difference.

Get out Never let a working week go by without doing something towards finding a new job. Every five days you should have made two positive efforts. These could include:

❖ Getting help to rewrite your CV
❖ Looking for job opportunities

- Applying for advertised jobs
- Writing to somewhere you would like to work
- Getting on a training course to help your employability

Get up If you can't get out, get up by getting promoted to a more challenging and interesting job. Use a five-weekly or even five-monthly ratio so that you don't irritate your bosses by constantly pushing for promotion, but definitely do two of the following:

- Let your boss know you are ready for something more challenging
- Look out for internal promotions
- Get noticed by volunteering for extra tasks
- Find ways to help your boss
- Network round the office with colleagues
- Resist the temptation to rush home, 'line-of-sight' delegation means you could get extra opportunities just by being there

Get on If this dull job really has your name on it, then on the positive side, you have the power to change it to make it more interesting. So for every five things that are tedious about your job, add or change two things to liven it up:

- Add extra elements, like creating an office newsletter
- Create a buzz by entering an office team in a fun run for charity

- ❖ Set up a lunchtime book club (you can be reading the book when you've run out of work tasks)
- ❖ Persuade your bosses to have a bring-your-child-to-work day
- ❖ Offer to mentor a work experience student
- ❖ If your firm gives you web access, learn a foreign language
- ❖ Join everything that's joinable

The formula for fitting in family life

Of all the issues people have with their work/life balance, fitting in family life is by far the most common. Surely it can't always have been like this? No, it wasn't always like this – it used to be worse! The balance between family life and work used to be achieved very simply by sending one parent (almost always the father) out to work and have the other parent (usually the mother) perform childcare. In some ways, this actually worked. Mums were always around to keep an eye on the children and they supported dads so that time could be spent at work without the need to worry about running the home.

But it was extremely inflexible. Social historians point out that the system left a lot of people very unhappy. Feminism tells us that it created misery for many go-getting women who would have liked to have had a career. What is less often highlighted is that society's expectations also gave men very little freedom of choice. If they wanted a family, they had to become a bread-winner, even if they might have longed to do something more creative but risky.

Today we have a lot more choice, and we should start thinking about our family/work balance with the knowledge that society in general is a lot more understanding about different lifestyles than it used to be. Stay-at-home dads; job shares; e-working; paternity leave; workplace nurseries – these are all possibilities that earlier generations didn't have. All we need to do is get organized, with the help of some balancing.

Can you have it all?

That's what we feel pressured to achieve. We are meant to be able to achieve career success; bring up happy children; keep fit and healthy; maintain a perfect marriage; and have a great social life. Steph is our test pilot for this area. Both she and her husband have high-profile careers, and their children are doing well at school. Steph is slim and gorgeous, and she and her husband are often to be seen enjoying their social lives together. So how come Steph instantly volunteered to become a test pilot when she heard I was researching the book?

Over a girly lunch she confessed: 'I sometimes feel like I need to get things under control. It can be a bit mad. I speak to the children via text. I think we sometimes do too much partying.'

If you can't have it all, have Five:Two

So if your attempts to 'have it all' are leaving you frazzled, try these techniques:

Prioritize Attempting to give every aspect of your life an equal amount of time and attention is impossible. Write a list of things that are going on in your life. It might read, in no particular order:

❖ Work
❖ Looking after my mum who's just moved in
❖ Hobby
❖ Spouse/partner
❖ Children
❖ Social life
❖ Trying to lose weight

Pick just two of those things to be your absolute priority. The other five will get attention, but they won't always be at the top of the list. Explain to your nearest and dearest that you are doing this, and tell them why. Ask for their help. You will be surprised. When they understand what's going on, family members can suddenly find ways of doing a lot more than they used to.

Compromise Once you have chosen your two priorities, accept that for a while you are going to miss out in other areas. If you usually take a couple of foreign holidays a year, but children and work are your two priorities, you have to accept a rather less glamorous life.

Analyse Choosing your priorities really gives you a chance to have a proper think about life. Keep revisiting your choices. They will change as you go on, so be adaptable.

Steph's Five:Two experience

Steph says: 'When I wrote all the elements down and thought about which two to prioritize, I realized it was a while since I'd done anything that was really about me. The family are all doing great, and I don't feel they need me so much. I want to take up horse riding again, and maybe re-evaluate my work.'

So Steph's list has self-development and hobby as the two priorities. She's going to discuss this with her husband so he knows she might not have so much time for socializing. She'll let us know how it goes.

The formula for the big break away

Sometimes your work/life balance needs a complete revamp, and this is where this formula can help. All you need to do is devote two sessions every five days towards your new work/life balance goal.

The moment for my big break away came when I was a busy senior executive on a national newspaper. I was trying to have it all and getting more exhausted every minute. Then I was asked to write a book about diet and lifestyle in my spare time, and realized I had no spare time. After a lot of soul searching, I understood that my work/life balance needed a complete change, and that's when I gave up the high-powered, but slightly lunatic world of daily newspapers and became a freelance author and journalist instead.

You may not need to go that far. 'Lifestyle working' is the new buzzword in business. It allows people to freshen up and rebalance their careers by opting for different work arrangements. Some companies have 'work-at-home-Wednesdays', others will offer different types of contract. It can be advantageous to both parties to re-employ you as a contractor or freelance. You can start researching these options in your two big-break sessions:

❖ Have a meeting with your HR department and ask about taking a short sabbatical – many firms now offer these, though you won't be on full pay while you are away.

❖ Check if there are any job-sharing schemes – again you may have to take a pay cut, but it might be worth it.

❖ Ask about e-working, and give some facts to back up your ideas about what you can do working online from home.

❖ Look around other companies in your line of work and see what sort of arrangements they have. You can either use this as a bargaining chip, or consider moving to a company with a better scheme.

The **Five:Two**
Relationships Plan

Working away from home? Long-distance love? Or just a tired old relationship routine? Using this plan can re-enliven relationships and help you through those difficult patches.

It's not only your significant other, though. Have you thought just how many relationships there are in your life? Have a quick count. As well as your spouse, partner or current special person, there may be children. Almost certainly relationships with mums, dads, sisters, brothers and even the extended family. Then there are your oldest friends from school and college. And your current social group, perhaps based around work or leisure pursuits. And your neighbours. What about your boss – that's a relationship too. And you may be responsible for juniors at work who report to you. Not forgetting the postman, or the lady you chat to at the bus stop most days, even though you haven't swapped names yet. And the other school-run mums and dads? And your children's teachers and friends – you should have a basic relationship, at least, with them.

There are also the relationships that are forced on you that you probably don't even think of as relationships. What about the chap at the phone company's call centre, who's terribly nice, but you can't understand a word he says – which wouldn't matter except that you've spent more time talking to him this week than you have to your husband. Like it or not, that's a relationship too!

Relationships with extroverts

Life is full of different relationships, all of which can go wrong from time to time. They also demand lots of our day-to-day energy. Sometimes the input from relationships is fantastic. Getting a phone call from a mate just when you're having a low moment can be all it takes to turn your mood right round.

There is a particular personality type called 'extrovert' who gets a lot of help from relationships. Extroverts are people who constantly look outwards towards their social circle, and that's where they get most of their emotional energy. If they are feeling low, they will go out for a drink or coffee with friends to cheer themselves up. They make great friends, and are often lively people – but they can be exhausting to have a relationship with. You can end up feeling as though you are always on call to help with any little crisis that may pop up into their lives. And sometimes, when you need a bit of support yourself, they are not fully there for you.

Relationships with introverts

The opposite personality type is an 'introvert' – someone who usually turns inwards when they are feeling low. When an introvert is worried or miserable, they will often curl up with a book or sit and think, rather than picking up the phone and chatting to a friend. On the whole, they don't need to get their emotional energy from outside, because they can find it within themselves.

Having a relationship with an introvert can be frustrating, because they are never going to be the first one to call and suggest lunch. You feel as if you are making all the running, and you may even be unsure whether they want to know you any more. Yet when you do get together for that lunch, your introvert friend usually proves to be a wonderful and sympathetic listener, and you go home feeling very re-energized.

The relationship two-way street

Emotional energy is a hugely important part of a relationship. Where both halves of the relationship have more-or-less balanced personalities, the energy flows both ways and the relationship is life-enhancing for both.

Where one or both of the halves has a very one-sided personality – very extrovert or very intro-vert – problems can crop up, because the energy ends up flowing only one way. Being in a relationship where the energy is only flowing one way – out of you and into

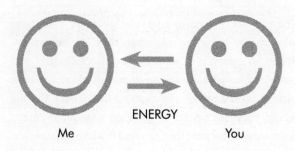

ENERGY

Me   You

the other person – is not only tiring, but also demoralizing and can eventually lead to real well-being and health issues. So it is important to be sure that you don't lose yourself in a relationship. Think of the relationship as being five Chunks for the other person and the relationship as a whole, with the other two Chunks being purely for yourself. Even at the start of a wonderful new relationship, where you may well be mad about the boy or the girl, remember to keep those two Chunks for yourself.

Relationship Rater

Do you constantly feel exhausted? Or slightly depressed? Do you never seem to have time to do anything for yourself? The answer could lie with your relationships. If you have one or more relationships where the energy is constantly flowing out of you and into the other person, you will soon start feeling down. And remember, it's not just your significant other relationship. This matters for all your relationships – with friends, bosses, family.

Which of your relationships feels like a one-way street? Test them out using this Relationship Rater. You can see on one side of the chart is your role in the relationship, and on the other side is their role. In between is the 'energy flow' section. Have a think about the relationship and work out which way the energy is flowing, then fill in an arrow to give the direction. If it's both ways, put two arrows in the two different directions. If it is maybe a lot one way, but also a little bit the other, put one arrow the whole way across the box, and the other just part way. Here's the box for my relationship with Steph:

Relationship Rater

Your Role	Energy Flow	Their Role
Old friend	$\longrightarrow$	Old friend
	$\longleftarrow$	

Oops! That already tells me I'm mainly on the receiving end in this relationship, so I'd better do something about it.

Mary filled in her flow chart for the main relationships in her life:

Relationship Rater

Your Role	Energy Flow	Their Role
Wife	→ ←	Husband
Mother	→ ←	Sons
Sister	→ ←	Brother
Daughter	→ ←	Father
Dog owner	←→	Dog
Colleague	→ ←	Colleague
Friend	→ ←	Friend
Neighbour	←→	Neighbour

Oh dear, it looks like Mary's most balanced relationship is with her dog! Well, they do say a dog is man's best friend. On the serious side, it is very easy to tell just from a glance at the arrows in the centre column how Mary is handling her relationships at the moment. In most of her relationships with men – husband, sons, father – Mary is the one putting the work in, and on the whole she's not getting much back. The most overlap is in the relationship with her husband, which is good news, but really it ought to be the full two-way street. In her relationship with her brother, it looks as if he is reaching out to her, but for some reason she isn't really responding very much. Mary might want to think about why that might be. And in her relationship with her father, there is a worrying gap between the two arrows, showing that there isn't very much emotional contact between them at all. A lot of this may be explained by looking at the arrows between Mary and her sons. It's easy to see that Mary is putting a huge amount of emotional energy into nurturing them, which is why she may not have much energy left for other relationships. And, as is the way with boys, there's not a lot coming back from them to her. That's fair enough. Children, and even young adults, should be secure enough to take their parents for granted. But the flip side of this is that it is up to us, as parents and grown-ups, not to take ourselves and our needs for granted.

Mary and I chatted about this. 'I see your point,' said Mary, 'but when the boys were younger and I was working full-time, I felt that they needed every bit of me that I could give. After all, I was at work so much of the time.'

'But, Mary, that was then. Now you are semi-retired and the youngest of the boys is at university. And isn't your oldest going to be thirty soon? Do you think it could be a habit you have got into, to have such an emotional one-way street between you and them?'

Mary doesn't agree about this, but one thing she does see as obvious is that she is giving out to men in general rather more than she is getting back. So Mary has decided to include this section on relationships in her programme and she will report back at the end.

Your Relationship Rater

Your Role	Energy Flow	Their Role

Women's Five and men's Two

Mary's experience of emotional energy flow in her relationships with men is not all that uncommon. It's widely believed that men are less committed to providing the energy a relationship needs than women are. In fact, this isn't really the case. The big difference is in the way the two sexes express themselves within a relationship.

By and large, women express themselves by talking . . . and then by talking . . . and maybe by having a glass of wine and talking some more. Whereas men are more like friendly dogs and express themselves by running about and wagging their tails. So if a man really wants to show his emotional attachment to a woman, he will do it physically in the first instance. A woman is more likely to show her love by saying it in words. Which is why we end up with women complaining: 'He's so insensitive' and men complaining: 'All she ever wants to do is talk.'

Women's Five is talking, and their Two is physical, but men's Five is physical, and their Two is talking. Yet this doesn't need to be a problem in a relationship – for many successful relationships it is actually a strength.

Match your moments

The first thing to do is accept that you're both different and match your 'talk:do' moments. Imagine you are about to take your dog for a walk. He's going to come bounding up and give you a thorough full-on physical expression of his devotion. That's fine, you expected that – and maybe even braced yourself if the dog is particularly large or bouncy. And off the two of you go for a lovely walk which you both enjoy without a word being said.

Now imagine you are going for lunch with an old friend. The waiter comes and goes three times before he manages to get your order because you have been chatting too much to look at the menu. You wouldn't take your dog out to lunch at a fancy restaurant, and you might not want to share a long wintry walk with your friend-who-lunches. It is pretty much the same in a male/female relationship, and for it to work well, you need to accept each other's Five:Two bias.

We are lucky that while dogs can't talk at all, men can. When it's important to talk, let the other half know that this is one of the times, but keep the whole balance of the relationship in proportion. You will find a balance that works in your relationship – for many conventional boy/girl relationships that may well end up being Five of doing, and Two of talking. Here are the main balances to remember in relationships:

Relationship balancers

❖ **Five for the relationship: Two for you** No matter how deeply engaged you are in a relationship, always retain your sense of self. Whether it is by doing two things on your own every week or by having two hours a day which are 'me time', keep hold of two for you.

❖ **Five of doing and showing: Two of talking** When it comes to deep emotions, our brains actually respond much better to the direct stimulation of doing and showing. Actions are felt to be more likely to be truthful, and speak more loudly than words. Save the talking for the more complex things.

❖ **Five of thinking first: Two of arguing** There are times when one party in a relationship needs to stand their ground and have a full-on row, but these times are much fewer than the actual occurrence of arguments. So think first before you fly off the handle.

❖ **Five in your boots: Two in their shoes** It can absolutely transform a relationship if you can put yourself into the other person's point of view. Even in the middle of a major row, try to imagine yourself in their shoes for a moment and actually believe their side of the argument. It can be hard to do, but makes a massive difference.

✤ **Five of moving on: Two of holding on** If things really have fallen apart, there comes a time to accept it and start rebuilding your world. It's all right to dwell on it a bit, but beware of letting it define your future.

The Five:Two Relationships Formulas

The formula for having a row

Yes, there is such a thing as a successful row – and there is a formula for it. For most of us, most of the time, a row is something that seems to blow up out of nowhere and run along uncontrollably like a sort of tornado, leaving a trail of broken furniture in its wake, sometimes literally. Some of us, particularly women, are so bothered by this that we avoid rows at all costs, surrendering on many fronts just to avoid a confrontation. Other people are self-confident enough to enjoy a bit of a row, especially making up afterwards, and it has to be admitted that these are more likely to be men.

If one person in the relationship is upset by rows, while the other half of the relationship sails through them, very quickly the relationship will become unbalanced, and eventually it will go downhill. The 'upset' party may appear to give in, but he or she will store up feelings of resentment. The 'oblivious' party will end up not getting any feedback at all, and much will go unsaid in the relationship that should have been brought out into the open. So occasional, positive rows are part of a healthy relationship. Here's how to manage a 'good' row, with two elements beforehand, and five things you should do during a row.

Before the row

Step One: Prepare

This may sound very strange, as almost by definition a row is an unexpected thing that you can't prepare for. Yet how many of your rows recently have been genuinely unexpected? If things are going through a sticky patch, you know there is a possibility you will end up in a row. Or if you want to raise a thorny problem, you have a feeling it may cause a row.

So be prepared, and learn to recognize quickly that a row is developing. As soon as you realize you are getting into a situation, switch into 'row alert mode'. Get all your troops mobilized and brace yourself so that you aren't taken by surprise by any storm tactics from the other side. The key thing is to look after yourself. A row is a war situation, even if only temporary. Keep reminding yourself: 'This is a row and I must keep myself safe.'

Step Two: Have an outcome in mind

The other important thing before a row starts is to have a very clear idea in your own mind what would be the ideal outcome of this row for you. Again, you may imagine that rows are too wild and uncontrollable to be able to do this. In fact, in most settled relationships, nearly all the rows are actually about the same problem – even though there may be different triggers for the row, the same old issue is nearly always at the bottom of it.

You know what your issues are. Think now, long before the next row, about exactly what those problems are. Work out what the ideal solution would be from your point of view. Ask yourself if that is really achievable? Now see if you can think of a compromise that would be acceptable for both of you.

That would be the outcome you want from the next row. You may not reach it soon, but it will make a huge difference to the way the row develops if you can keep a strong grip on that positive outcome that you might both want, no matter what is said during the row. It might help to write yourself a short note of your positive outcome.

During the row

Tactic One: Deal with your own anger

This is a row, it's normal to be angry. Yet at the same time, if you are going to have a successful outcome to your row, you need to stay in control of things. So it's important not to let your anger control you. If you can, try to stand aside from your anger. By all means, let it go – it can be a very useful weapon – but don't let it prevent you from thinking clearly and pursuing your row tactics. Imagine you are a general in command of his troops in battle. The general has to stay calm and organize everything while the heavy artillery is firing all round. Be your own general.

Tactic Two: Don't whinge

Meaningless whingeing won't get you anywhere in a row. Stick to your point, keep your outcome in mind, and don't waste your ammunition on a host of minor irritations. If you have done your pre-row preparation, you are ideally positioned to take the high ground in this row. In other words, both sides will know in their heart of hearts that you are actually in the right. Whingeing defeats this. Banging on and on about 'another thing' just makes you sound petty.

Tactic Three: Mirroring

This is a very powerful tactic used by professional interviewers. You act as a 'mirror' to the other side of the row. You can do it in two ways – body language and words. Many of us unconsciously mirror the body language of someone we are chatting with, particularly if we feel a strong bond. If the other person rests their chin on their hand, or crosses their legs, we can adopt the same position. Because it's a signal that the subconscious mind recognizes as friendly, then this body language mirroring can be a good way to defuse a row that is getting out of hand. Be careful how you use it. If the other person becomes aware that you are doing this deliberately they will find it irritating.

The other mirroring tactic is to say back to someone what they have just said to you. Your co-rower might say:

'I'm so fed up with you for forgetting to fill the car up with petrol again.' You can reply: 'I can understand that you're cross with me for forgetting to fill the car up.' This is such a positive tool to use in a row. It recognizes that the other person has a legitimate complaint, which makes them feel good. On the other hand, you haven't actually apologized yet (although it might be on your agenda), and you are opening the way for you to have a right of reply, which might go like this: 'I can understand that you're cross with me for forgetting to fill up the car, and I'm sorry for that, because I know it's irritating. There is a reason. Can I tell you why that happened?' Now, while the other side is feeling a bit better because you have mirrored, is your chance to get your own point across.

Tactic Four: Changing sides

This is a useful tactic for using when a row is getting out of hand. For a moment, just switch sides. So instead of arguing your point, adopt the other person's point of view. This certainly takes the wind out of their sails, since it needs two to make a row. It has the effect of slowing the whole row down for a while and giving you both a breather. Another benefit is that while you are 'on their side' you do get a chance to see things from their point of view, and that can often help you both to reach agreement in the end.

Tactic Five: Steer the row

This element is really the overall effect that you will achieve if you prepare properly and then use the right tactics throughout the row. You will find that you can steer the row in the direction you want it to go. Rather than being on the back foot all the time, reacting and responding to the challenges from the other person, you are the one taking the lead. This is being 'pro-active' – taking the battle to the enemy. Keep in mind the outcome you planned in preparation, and use all your tactics throughout the row to steer it towards that outcome. Once you get the hang of this, your co-rower may even feel they have 'won' the row. In fact, you will both have achieved a mutually acceptable outcome.

The formula for breaking up

A great friend of mine isn't a particularly good listener to other people's moans about relationship break-ups. She lets you run on for a while, before fixing you with a charming but meaningful look and saying: 'But you're over it now.' Sure enough, you have to acknowledge that she's right really – and if you aren't over it, you certainly should be.

It doesn't really matter who caused the break-up, both sides are likely to feel there is some unfinished business. This is where things can get messy and dangerous. Post break-up contact leads to recriminations and soon a new negative 'broken-up' relationship has formed. We all know such situations. Where celebrities or politicians are concerned they often hit the headlines, as both parties engage in revenge campaigns against each other.

Revenge is a dish best not served at all. Revenge always rebounds on the vengeful one, often having bounced off the other party with them barely having noticed. Trying to take revenge is the biggest signal of all that you are not over it. So here are the five dos and two don'ts for moving on after the end of a relationship:

- ✓ **Do** take charge of your own life
- ✓ **Do** rediscover yourself as an individual
- ✓ **Do** make a calm, sensible plan for any residual matters about the relationship (belongings etc.)
- ✓ **Do** stay in touch with friends from both sides of the old relationship
- ✓ **Do** hand everything over to a neutral party (e.g. a lawyer) if the ex is showing signs of being vengeful
- ✗ **Don't** try to take revenge on your ex
- ✗ **Don't** bitch about your ex to other people

The formula for reigniting a rocky relationship

The most common advice given to couples hitting a rough patch is: 'Go for a long weekend in the country together.' Which is the worst possible thing you could do. If you are bored with each other now, you are going to be doubly bored with each other in some empty, out-of-season country hotel. If you are rowing with each other, the last place to do it is in public, in a fancy restaurant.

Couples would probably do better to go for a long weekend in the country *without* each other, or even with someone else, like a friend. Other techniques often advised can actually have rather comical results. Massaging each other with oil is all very well if you are young things passionately in love. For a middle-aged couple who haven't been relaxedly intimate since the birth of their first child, the whole oil and candles thing is just desperately embarrassing and stressful.

In many ways it's best to do as little as possible. If the relationship is feeling fragile, taking on new activities together can feel very pressurizing. So the trick is to back off a bit. First of all, keep faith in the relationship. Trust it to totter along until times are better. Give each other some space. If you are rowing all the time, follow the row formula. If you are bored with each other, that could be because you are spending too much time together, rather than too little. Bored people are often boring people. So find individual interests that you can do separately.

At the beginning of the relationship, five Chunks of your energy are devoted to the relationship, and two to yourself. When a relationship is creaking, it is time to flip Five:Two over, and put five Chunks of energy into yourself, and two into the relationship. Once you are both starting to feel sufficiently confident in yourselves as individuals again, then it is time to re-meet each other. Ask one another on dates – first one person fixes the date, and then the other. The date might be to ask the other half to join you on one of your new activities.

Remember, when you first met each other you were complete strangers, yet you eventually fell in love. Each of you will have changed a lot during the course of the relationship, and now is the time to honour that. Rediscover the stranger in each other. It's very exciting, like having an affair, but without the risks!

The **Five:Two**
Beat the Years Plan

Are you starting to feel older? Well, of course we can't avoid that – ageing is a fact of life. In fact, the whole population of the UK, and the world, is ageing. As we all begin to live longer, and fewer people die young, so the average age of the population is increasing. At the moment, one in six people in Britain is aged sixty-five or over, and that will gradually increase to a quarter of the population in the next thirty to forty years.

So if you are beginning to feel a bit older, you're in good company – so is everyone. There's no need to think you are the only one it's happening to. With more and more of us in the over-fifties and over-sixties bracket, it means that being older is going to get very trendy. Life will actually become easier, as services and consumerism are targeted at older people. The other good news is that there are not just more of us, we are also individually living to an older age. Average life expectancy is increasing even more rapidly than scientists expected. According to the UK Office for National Statistics, women are now living to an average age of 82.8 years and men 78.8 years. This is already an increase of more than a year in little over a decade.

What does that mean to you as an individual?

You're likely to be living a lot longer than your parents' generation, and so will those around you, which means we are all going to have to rethink our ideas about 'old age'. What is old now? My grandfather was born to a poor family in 1890, when average life expectancy was just forty-four years. He left school at eleven years old and suffered from a deprivation-related disease, rickets. Yet he lived to be ninety-eight years of age. For me, growing up with all the advantages of modern health care, it looks as if I should bargain on living to 100 and beyond. So, even though at fifty-five, I'm beginning to feel a bit of a wrinkly, I'd better get over it, because I'm only halfway through my life!

What's the point of living longer?

Now we've all got over the excitement of being just spring chickens in our fifties and sixties, it's time to start thinking about how we are going to enjoy those extra ten or twenty years we can look forward to. What's bothering researchers is the possibility that we might end up spending those years sitting in a chair being ill, miserable and dependent.

HALE: Healthy Active Life Expectancy

There really isn't any point living more years unless you are healthy and happy enough to enjoy them. Over the last fifteen or twenty years researchers, including those at Oxford University's 'Healthy Ageing Project', have developed the idea of HALE: Healthy Active Life Expectancy. This means that instead of just adding years to our life, we are also going to put some life in our years. The Oxford University researchers want us to have the fullest possible lives right up to the very last moment, just like my grandfather did.

Put the life into your years

The picture that many people have of old age as something negative is completely wrong, say the researchers. We can be running marathons or flying microlight aircraft (like Wing Commander Ken Wallis from the James Bond movies who died at the age of ninety-seven still holding eight world records) into our nineties. There's no need at all to be sitting in a chair staring at the telly all day long. And the most recent studies are proving them right.

The Swedish study

Researchers at Sweden's Karolinska Institute (one of Europe's largest and most prestigious medical universities) discovered in 2012 that being active, and living a healthy lifestyle, into your seventies can add six years to your life. They found that men and women who took up activities like swimming or walking increased their life expectancy by around two years. And people with a busy social life lived more than a year longer than those without. When they combined the figures for those who adopted the most healthy options all round, the researchers were amazed to discover that men could extend their lives by six years, and women by five years.

In Britain, Professor Alan Maryon-Davis, professor of public health at King's College, London, believes: 'These results should put an extra spring in the step of everyone in later life. They provide good evidence that even in your seventies it's not too late to gain an extra few years to enjoy life by keeping active, living healthily and being involved in family and community.'

And it's never too late

The Swedish researchers were particularly excited to find that the healthy activity formula worked even for those who hadn't been leading healthy lifestyles when younger. They knew that being sedentary, overweight, a smoker, or heavy drinker is bad for health and shortens life expectancy. But surprisingly, they also found that those who improved their lifestyles in middle age, by giving up smoking for example, were almost as long-lived as those who had never smoked. So it is never too late to start looking after your health.

HALE – and hearty

If that hasn't cheered you up already, here's another ageing statistic that gives an upbeat picture of what we have to look forward to: the Office for National Statistics surveyed happiness in Britain in 2013, and found that people aged fifty-five and older are the most contented group. So there's every reason to have a really positive attitude to getting older. Yet so many of us dread those first few grey hairs; the aches and pains that come from nowhere; the worries about being out of touch when your year of birth is further and further down the drop-down list. Five:Two is here to help with all those worries, and show you that they can all be beaten!

We now know that it is medically and scientifically proven that we not only can, but should, go on having just as much fun as we did when younger, if not more. Why then, do you hear so many self-limiting remarks: 'Oh, I can't possibly do that at my age.' Or: 'I'm afraid I can't do the walking any more because of my feet.' And often people say things like: 'I would have loved to go to the party, but I don't hear very well now, so it's a bit difficult.'

Invisible agers

We tend to accept the things we associate with old age as being inevitable – and incurable. I call these the 'Invisible Agers'. My research with doctors specializing in gerontology (the study of old age) has shown me that these 'Invisible Agers' are both avoidable and curable. It's time to get tough! Don't put up with bad feet, aching bones and difficulty in reading small print. Do something about it – now.

The trouble is that if you don't do something about your Invisible Agers now, they will gradually creep up on you and get you in the end. One doctor told me about a patient of his who was in a poor state, even though as a young woman she had been a very popular dancer. What happened was that she had developed terrible bunions and corns. Gradually her feet had become so painful that she was hardly walking at all. She gained weight and didn't go out of the house very much, eventually becoming rather depressed. The doctor saw her when she had fallen downstairs and broken her hip. Because of lack of the 'sunshine' vitamin D which your body gets from being outdoors, and lack of weight-bearing exercise (combined with menopause), she had developed osteoporosis – a disease which makes the bones very brittle. The doctor told me: 'All this could have been prevented if she'd only had her feet sorted out at the beginning when they first started hurting.'

Beat the invisible agers

There is so much you can do now that will transform your life, not only in the present, but for the whole of your future. Top up your full spectrum (outdoors) light for just two days a week and your vitamin D levels will soon be high enough to help fight age-related fatigue and bone-thinning. Do weight training just two hours a week and you can defeat the onset of osteoporosis. The body's natural rhythms work on a Five:Two cycle, so adjusting your beauty regime to fit will have successful results. Even if you're not getting your beauty sleep you can still use this cycle to get the rest and refreshment you need.

Now check out the invisible agers and what to do about them, and discover your Two Secret Weapons:

Five Invisible Agers

1. **Foot pain** – Get into the habit of going to a proper chiropodist (not a beauty pedicure) regularly to stop corns, bunions etc. before they become a problem.
2. **Vision problems** – Don't accept failing vision: go to the optician. It is very important to continue being able to read easily in order to keep your brain active and prevent age-related decline in faculties (Alzheimer's etc.).
3. **Hearing impairment** – Often this can be transformed just by your local nurse giving your ears a thorough cleanse. And there are new cures for more serious hearing problems. As soon as you notice a decline, get it checked.

4. **Isolation** – During ageing, the less we do, the less we will be able to do, causing a downward spiral which scientists call 'morbidity'. So make a conscious effort to get out and about as much as, or more than, you did ten years ago.

5. **Dependency** – It really is a case of 'use it or lose it' as we get older. It's wonderful when people want to help, but remember you are a grown-up and you will be surprised at how much you can do for yourself.

Two Secret Weapons

1. **Optimism** – Look at the people you know or see in the media who are doing fabulously in old age. Believe that you can be like them. Ageing is about second chances. Now is the time in your life to do the things you never quite got round to when you were too busy or didn't have the opportunity.

2. **Self-help** – The more stuff you can do for yourself, the longer you will go on doing stuff. Only you know what Invisible Agers you are feeling, so only you can do something about them.

> Turn your I wishes into I wills

Five:Two For Anti-Ageing

The different formulas below are designed to solve the main issues we all face with ageing, and some will speak to you more than others. For example, if you had a relative who suffered from age-related mental problems like confusion or even Alzheimer's, you may be worried about keeping your brain working well, so the formula for mental sharpness will be ideal.

If it's the grey hairs and wrinkles that bother you, the formula for looks has plenty of tips for turning back the years. Whatever our personal concerns, all of us will benefit from following some or all of the formulas. Use this opportunity to give yourself a fifty-plus MOT check, and then start resetting your ageing clock.

> Five days of routine
> Two days of anti-ageing action

Before you get started on formulas, time to find out what your life expectancy is now, and what you could do to change it.

Life-Expectancy Chart

Starter years: 80		+ Yrs		− Yrs	Fill in your running total below:
Things you can't change:	Female	+2	Male	−2	
	Under 50	+2	Over 50	−2	
	Grandparent still alive	+1			
	Mother lived beyond 80	+1			
			Family history of heart disease or cancer	−2	
	Living in south of UK	+1	Living in north of UK	−1	
Things you can change:	Non-smoker	+0	Smoker	−2	
			Diabetes	−4	
			Heart disease	−2	
	Normal weight	+1	Overweight	−1	
	Exerciser	+2	Non-exerciser	−1	
	Graduate	+2	Non-graduate	+0	
	Hobbies	+1			
	Active social life	+1			
Approximate life expectancy:					

What's your life expectancy?

Assuming a typical life expectancy of eighty years, this life-expectancy chart shows what you can do to increase that figure, and the health and lifestyle issues that will decrease it. Fill in each block and keep the running total, and you will find your personal life expectancy at the end.

Now fill your chart in again, but this time change the things you could change, like becoming a non-smoker or reversing diabetes, and see the difference in your life expectancy.

Five things to do now to increase your HALE

1. Start moderate exercise outdoors (check out the Fitness Plan)
2. Join a club
3. Take up a new hobby
4. Cook and eat healthy food
5. Challenge yourself

Two things to stop doing

1. Stop being overweight
2. Stop smoking

Beat The Years Formulas

The formula for mental sharpness

Do you find it hard to understand the instructions when you get a new phone? Are you having trouble catching up with what people are talking about? The good news is, this may be nothing at all to do with your brain, and everything to do with poor sight and poor hearing. You can't understand the phone instructions because the print is too small to read. And you don't catch what people are saying because you have a mild hearing problem. So get those Invisible Agers sorted out. The best way of staying sharp right into old age is to put your brain to work. Research has found those who regularly do word and number puzzles have quicker brains. Make sure that the puzzles are tough enough; aim to get to the next level every time you play.

It has recently been discovered that you can really get your brain firing on all cylinders by doing mental activity at the same time as physical activity. Think chess boxing! Yes, chess boxing really is a sport. The competitors each make a move on the chess board, which is next to the boxing ring, then spar for a minute, before rushing back to the board for the next move. I have tried it, and can report that by the third or fourth round, you are so mentally and physically exhausted you can barely even remember your name.

You don't have to go that far, but you could try running through your multiplication tables or the kings and queens of England, the next time you are out for a jog. At the gym, get your training partner to fire mental arithmetic questions at you while you are weight training. The formula is to use five Chunks of brain power, balanced with two Chunks of exercise, as much as you can. Introduce as much new stimulation for your brain as possible. So every five days, ask your brain two new questions. You could learn your seventy-five times table. You could use the internet to research something you've always wanted to know about. It doesn't always have to be serious stuff. Get your grandchildren to test you on names of boy-band members. The aim is to get your brain to keep sparking, and to fire up as many new areas as possible.

Every time you have a new thought, or solve a problem, your brain has to make a new connection between different cells. How about finding out how this actually works? During the thinking process neuro-transmitters (biological chemicals) transmit signals from neurons (electrically sensitive nerve cells in your brain) across a little gap called a synapse to reach a new 'target' cell, so that a new pathway is formed between the two – which makes the thinking capacity of your brain bigger. There are now brain scanners which can actually show this process happening and it is stunningly beautiful, like a firework display in your brain, triggering activity to glow and fade and glow again. You can have your own firework display in your head, and the more rockets that go off, the sharper your brain will remain.

The formula for looking after yourself

As trainee journalists on local newspapers, one of the fun jobs we had to do was interview 100-year-olds on their birthday. After they'd shown us their card from the Queen, we always had to ask: 'So how have you lived to be a hundred?' The answer was always the same: 'A little bit of what you fancy does you good.' The number of great-grans I've met who put away a tot or two of whisky or port every evening would surprise you. My own grandfather was the same. He bought good red wine by the half-bottle, and had a glass every evening with his dinner. Since these half bottles were not intended for sharing, this didn't always go down too well with the family, who would grumble about him 'looking after himself'.

He got it right – older age is the time in your life to put yourself first. After a lifetime of working and childcare, this really is your time. All too often though, we're very out of practice at looking after ourselves. So here are five steps you can take to look after yourself, and two lovely rewards.

Step One: The fifty-plus MOT test

Treat yourself like a classic car and put yourself through a simple fifty-plus MOT test. If you fail any of the checks, make sure you get it put right, just as you would with a car. There are tests for: sight, hearing, diabetes, cholesterol and fitness.

Step Two: Me moments

Make sure you have a 'Me Moment' every day, whether it is a nice glass of wine, or watching your favourite soap, or a long, hot soak in the bath. The older you get, the more Me Moments you deserve. You can have 'Me Days' as well!

Step Three: Get me everybody

Worries as you get older can drag you downhill. If you have a particular problem, like worries about heating the house, or what pensions you are due, remember there is plenty of free help and advice around. You can share these worries with professionals whose job it is to help you. All it takes is a phone call, or an email. There are some contact details at the back of this book, but the simplest and easiest way to get help with these issues is to tell your doctor about them. She won't mind and she will be able to put you in touch with the right people to help.

Step Four: My hobby

One of the huge plus points of retiring is that you finally get time for your own interests. If you've had to put it on hold in the past, now is the time to take up your favourite hobby again. For probably the first time in your life, you can make it one of your main priorities. So if you used to enjoy walking, organize a long-distance walk to go on. If you used to garden, see if you can get or share an allotment. Many sixty-plus people suddenly find their hobby turns into a second post-retirement career. My neighbour has now become a very successful professional market gardener, supplying our local farm shop.

Step Five: My family

Yes, they come as the last step! We put our families first for most of our lives, but it's not necessary to do so for ever. It's all too easy to become entangled in grandparenting and even great-grandparenting, particularly as so many families need help with childcare and even housing. If you love it, and it keeps you feeling young, great. However, it's not for everybody, and you shouldn't feel guilty if you want your post-retirement years to be a time for you and your partner to strike out on your own.

Reward One: Rediscover yourself

Once you are able to go through all your five steps successfully, you will probably be surprised to find that instead of shutting down as you feared, your later life is opening up in front of you. Any health problems are under control. You are enjoying some well-earned treats. You have found professional help with money and similar worries. You are finally getting round to things you always meant to do. And hopefully the family has come to terms with the fact that you are no longer an unpaid servant. The day you tick all those boxes is the day you rediscover yourself – or even discover a brand-new self.

Reward Two: Enjoy your freedom

Celebrate the new – or even old – you by having some fun. Find your funny bone again and do silly things for the sheer hell of it. Add up the ages of your social set and have a joint 215th birthday party, or whatever it comes to. A really important part of looking after yourself is not taking yourself too seriously.

The formula for looks

Sometimes it really does seem like old age has got it in for us, especially when it comes to the way our looks change. The greying hair, the wrinkles, the sagging skin and loss of muscle tone hit both men and women. But we can't all be George Clooneys and Helen Mirrens. Or can we? If you learn to work with the changes brought by age, you can still feel great about yourself, and look great too. Eve Pollard, British broadcaster and self-confessed 'grumpy old woman', says that she and her female friends of a certain age have all 'gone prematurely blonde'. She's right – if you've been a mouse or a brunette all your life, those grey hairs are going to give your hairdresser a chance to make you blonder than ever!

Five very simple ways to keep age at bay

1. **Work out with weights** Research has shown that exercising with weights is a great way of preventing one of the biggest ageing problems, osteoporosis, and it is also a great looks enhancer. When you are younger your skin is supported by collagen, as well as a little fat under the skin, called subcutaneous fat. As you get older you lose both of these, which is why your skin ends up saggy and less elastic. Pumping up the muscles underneath your skin will do some of that work, and give the same plump, taut effect that younger skin naturally has.

2. **Love your skin** Ageing skin needs more tlc, but it responds very well. You don't need expensive anti-ageing creams. Just drink lots of fluids (water, juice) to keep your skin plump and hydrated. Exfoliate every time you wash. On your body you can do this using a soft-bristled body brush to remove dead skin cells. Be more gentle with your face and use a muslin cloth or oatmeal. After cleansing and exfoliating, massage in a simple oil-based moisturizer and finish with a blob of sunscreen.

3. **Make-up** Not only does your face shape change as you age, so does your complexion. This means that colours which suited you ten years ago might be too harsh now. And the style of make-up you use will have to adapt as well. The simplest way to get on top of this is to get a free make-over at the beauty counter of your nearest department store.

4. **Embrace your age** Mutton dressed as lamb is one thing, but mutton dressed as a foxy vixen is quite another. Look your own age rather than trying to get away with ten years younger, and you will look great no matter what. That might mean covering up a cleavage that has seen too much sun, but it doesn't stop you wearing a fantastic pair of shoes.

5. **Renew your wardrobe** The most reviving thing you can do for yourself is chuck out half your wardrobe. Those jeans you have been trying to slim into for the past three years, accept that you are not now going to be able to slim into them. Editing your wardrobe may also give you a chance to rediscover

some wonderful vintage pieces that are now timeless classics. Take them to a good dry cleaner and have them brought back to life, but don't let your daughter or granddaughter get hold of them or you'll never get them back.

And two things not to do:

1. **Don't smoke** Regardless of the health issues, smoking is the most ageing thing you can possibly do to your looks. If you have a non-smoking friend your age, compare the backs of your hands and you will see. Smoking literally kippers your face and hands, causing wrinkles, discolouration and loss of suppleness. Buying anti-ageing skin cream is a waste of time if you are a smoker.

2. **Don't get too thin** – The leading French dermatologist Dr Jean Sebagh has a massive list of celebrity clients in both America and France. His main piece of advice is free: 'Most of my female clients are a few pounds too thin which means that the skin is more prone to be loose.' So one of the plus points of ageing is that you no longer have to chase down that last half stone, because you will look more youthful with it than without it.

The formula for positive energy

The great thing about ageing today is that there are so many extraordinary sexy and exciting examples of sixty-plus people and celebrities getting out there and enjoying life no matter what. Felicity Kendal doing a yoga class has got my personal trainer in a bit of a state, while I must confess to a bit of a hankering after Hugh Cornwell (once lead singer of The Stranglers), even after all he's been through! Which is rather the point. When Johnny Depp (by the way, a mid-lifer himself) was looking for inspiration for the famously charismatic pirate Captain Jack Sparrow, it was Keith Richards who provided the necessary shot of cool – though of course Jack is never quite as cool as his dad.

Ageing is cool, and it is going to get super-cool. As the population gets older, what older people do by definition will be the trendy thing to do, just because there are more of us doing it. So whatever it is you feel like doing, do it. Do do *something*, though.

The challenge

Researchers into ageing, and especially maintaining mental sharpness into old age, have found that having new experiences is the best way to keep the mind and spirit young. So challenge yourself. Aim to have two new big adventures every five years from now on. It doesn't matter what the adventure is, as long as it's something a little outside your comfort zone. So if you have always holidayed in a hotel or resort, challenge yourself to go camping instead. Buy a bike and learn to cycle. It could be something you've always wanted to do but never got

round to. In my teens and twenties I was a bit of a swot –
it wasn't until I was in my fifties that I went to my first
rock concert.

Here's a planner chart for you to fill in to make your
own Life List.

Your Life List

What I wish I could do	What I'm going to do	When I'm doing it	Done it!

The **Five:Two** Partying and Social Media Plan

Is the social whirl getting too much? Have those drinks on a Friday night turned into a seven-night marathon? This book will show you how to create a new healthy regime to eliminate the bad effects of too much partying, and help you manage your social drinking and behaviour in the future.

Recovery is reachable

Luckily for us, our body is amazingly resilient to much of the worst we can throw at it. Our livers, for example, can regrow to compensate for as much as seventy-five per cent liver damage. If the damage is only mild, just a couple of weeks of no drinking will enable your liver to get back in shape. It is the same with smoking. After only twelve hours of quitting, your blood oxygen level increases to normal, and carbon monoxide levels go back down to where they should be. And it just gets better.

By the time you have stopped smoking for a whole year, your lungs will be functioning properly, and a whole host of illness risks will have decreased dramatically.

Clinical research has shown how the body can be helped into rapid, healthy recovery from even quite serious addiction problems. So whether you are just pushing it a bit too much, or you suspect you may have a real problem, it is *always* worth trying to do something about it.

The new temptations

Most of us are well aware of the risks of the major life-threatening addictions: drugs, alcohol and tobacco. They have been with us for a long time. There is evidence that very early civilizations used all three. Today though, in the space of a single lifetime, a whole new range of tempting, but possibly unhealthy activities have sprung up. Home television sets became widely available only in the late 1950s, but now at least eighty per cent of homes all over the world have TV sets, and it has transformed the way people live.

Brave new world?

In only the last few years, we've also got tablets, mobile phones, laptops and all sorts of other digital devices.

We are connected twenty-four/seven, wherever we go, whatever we are doing. Is this always a good thing? Psychologists are beginning to think not. Researchers have discovered that getting a text or being tweeted prompts our brains to produce a chemical called dopamine, which is one of the body's 'feel-good' substances. So every time a new media message pings into our lives it gives us an emotional buzz. This mini-high becomes addictive, and can lead to an obsessive need to check social media. One doctor even recommends her patients to have an 'electronic sundown' ninety minutes before bed, with no technology.

Do you constantly feel 'wired not tired' at the end of the day? Are you addicted to your mobile? Do you tweet more than is good for you? Or are you fanatical about Facebook? This book has a simple technique for breaking addictions to social media and television, without having to give up the fun completely.

Addictive personalities

Some addictions are more obviously destructive than others, but in fact all addictions have a lot in common. It is not unusual for someone to suffer from more than one addiction. This is called multiple addiction, and psychologists have identified an 'addictive personality', which they believe is more likely to be unable to stop within safe limits.

A lot of people can have a drink fairly regularly, and even overdo it once in a while, without things getting out of control. They wake up with a hangover, think 'never again', and probably go on the wagon for a couple of weeks. But addictive personality types find this impossible. Even though they wake feeling awful, having more alcohol is so important that they somehow manage to convince themselves either that the alcohol wasn't the cause of feeling awful, or that it won't be the same next time.

Inheriting an addictive personality

The statistics show that the children of addicts are much more likely to become addicts themselves. Scientists aren't quite sure whether this is because of an inherited genetic problem, or because children of addicts are brought up to accept addiction. But the sad fact is that it does increase risk. Melanie, one of our control test group, told me why she is so careful to maintain a healthy lifestyle: 'My mother was addicted to alcohol and smoking, but my dad is the opposite. He can have a drink at a party and then not drink for days. Before the smoking ban he was the same with cigarettes. He would have one after a meal, and then completely forget about smoking. I think I take after my father, but I'm careful to keep exercising just the same.'

But there are all sorts of other addictions apart from alcohol and cigarettes. I wish Melanie was one of the test pilots. She goes out for a drink with friends most nights, but assumes exercising every day is a compensation. Could the amount of exercise she does be an addiction in itself? And is she sure that drinking most nights isn't pushing outside the safety zone?

What's your scale?

Imagine Melanie's dad is one out of ten on the addictive scale, and her mother is nine out of ten. Where would you put Melanie on the scale? And now, the big question: Where would you put yourself? That can be a hard question to answer. When is spending a couple of hours gaming an OK amount of time? How long do you have to be doing it before it is too much? And how about if your gaming spills over into gambling websites? It may be only a few pounds a week now, but what if it rose to be more than you could really afford?

Asking your nearest and dearest what they think isn't always helpful. You may not like the answer. You really have to ask yourself these questions. Again, you may not like the answer. The fact that you are reading this section certainly points to there being some issue somewhere.

Asking the hard questions

But do you really have an addiction? Or is it simply that you need to get some of the less healthy aspects of your lifestyle under control? That really is the big question. Health professionals have known for a long time that those most in need of help are the ones least likely to ask for it. Addicts are often in denial about their addiction. For all of us it can be very hard to confront the truth that we might be harming ourselves through our lifestyles. The really positive thing in all this is that doctors and psychologists agree that admitting the truth, and facing up to it, is the biggest and most important step anyone can take towards getting better.

Let's face it

So now it's time to ask ourselves those hard questions. Below are some little stories, scenarios, of everyday events. The way we react to those situations can tell us a lot about how addicted we might be. Like all the questionnaires in this book, there are no right or wrong answers, just honest ones. In this case, almost more than any other, it's important to be honest with yourself. Make a note of your reaction to each event described, and you will find it very revealing.

Happy-hour scenario

You are just about to pour yourself that pre-dinner glass of wine or gin and tonic that you have been looking forward to. You certainly feel you deserve it. Then the phone rings and it's your daughter's school explaining that transport from the gym club has had to be cancelled and they are asking parents to come and collect their children. What next? Do you grumpily put down the bottle, knowing that you have to fetch your daughter, but feeling very resentful that your glass of wine will have to wait an hour? Or perhaps you have a quick half-glass and then set off? Maybe you wouldn't even consider that; instead you dash out to the car to pick up your daughter, completely forgetting about the drink you had been looking forward to. Or do you have a quick ring round of other mums to see if they can give your daughter a lift so you can have that drink in peace? And here is another thought: could it be that actually, this isn't going to be your first drink of the day? Maybe you had a couple of drinks at lunchtime. Is there a possibility that you may already be over the legal limit for driving?

Melanie is the one who came up with this scenario. She emailed me: 'This did happen to me quite a few times when I was at school. Usually I would try to get buses home, which was a bit tricky as we weren't on a bus route. It was only when I grew up that I realized my mother hadn't been able to collect me because of drinking.'

138

Think about your answers

Which of the reactions is closest to yours? It isn't difficult to see where your answers are pointing. If you instantly put your daughter's needs first and completely forget about drinking, then you have no problems. Most of us would probably put our daughter first and be a bit grumpy – again, not really an issue. But any of the answers where the alcohol basically comes ahead of your daughter in your priorities shows that you do have a problem. And that problem could be really serious.

> **Face it**: If you are already over the drink–drive limit at five or six o'clock on a weekday evening, you have an alcohol problem. The place to deal with that problem is with your doctor. Put this book down and make an appointment. Now.

Career scenario

You have a very important job interview in the morning and you will need to get up early and be on your best form, especially as it's a job you really want. What's the plan? Do you make sure you get an early night, even though it means missing a really good Sunday-nighter gig? Do you not make any plans and just assume it will work out OK? Or maybe you go out as normal, but set your alarm just to be on the safe side. Do you even go full-on clubbing and turn up at the interview without having slept?

This scenario happened to our test pilot Mark, who is just finishing his course at university. He admitted: 'Yeah, big no-no. I had an interview for an internship, went out just for a couple of beers, ended up going on clubbing then missed the alarm in the morning.' So although socializing with mates sounds completely harmless, it can easily tip over into being a problem in your life.

Missed-opportunity scenario

You are really stuck into the latest release of your special online game, in the middle of a massive action scene. The phone rings and it's a friend with a spare ticket to see your favourite band, who you've always wanted to see live, but you'll need to catch the train more or less now to get there in time. Do you drop everything and get out the door, even though it means you will lose your chance to win the online battle and get up to the next level? Do you spend some time saving your position and then rush off, hoping you'll still be able to catch the train? Perhaps you regretfully tell your friend to give the ticket to someone else so you can go on playing. Or maybe you never even answered the phone in the first place, so you will never know what it might have been.

Thinking about this situation, you can see whether your gaming has reached the point where it is actually dominating your life. If you wouldn't have answered the phone, who knows what wonderful real-life opportunities for adventure and personal growth you are missing out on.

Peer-pressure scenario

One of your friends has got a troll on Twitter and she's really upset by it. The problem is you know who the troll is, and it is one of your close friends. But the troll has got a great network and she's friended you into some brilliant areas. Do you go along with the troll and even re-tweet? Or do you stand up for your friend against the troll, even though it means you might lose out? Perhaps you go as far as telling your friend who the troll is. Maybe you would like just to shut down those networks, so you can stay out of it, but you feel you can't, in case you miss out on stuff being said to or about you.

This scenario describes one of the biggest issues with social media that psychologists are worried about. Bullying will always be a fact of life, particularly among teenagers. What bothers teachers and doctors is that bullying through social media is much harder to deal with. It can spread virally to a huge network of people. Adults are involved in social-media bullying as much as children. There is no face-to-face contact, so the bullies can hide behind their anonymity. And many people feel

compelled to side with the bully because of peer pressure –
that understandable desire to stay part of the gang.

Now choose your formula

Looking at the scenarios above will have given you a
much better self-knowledge about your own particular
issues – whether it's alcohol or clubbing or media-
related. So now choose your formula. But first, please
read this note.

Important Medical Note on
Clinical Addictions

Some addiction and overuse problems are
an immediate danger to your health. These
addictions need professional help. If you think
you may be suffering from clinical addiction,
please seek medical help. If you are trying to
give up smoking or drugs, you need to contact
a professional organization. These plans are
not suitable for those wishing to give up
smoking or drugs and are not suitable for
addressing clinical addiction.

The Five:Two partying and social media formulas

The formula for drink control

It's so exciting to realize that the principles of Five:Two apply really well to getting your drinking back in balance. The method actually works with your body's own natural cycles of self-healing. The liver needs two weeks to recover from moderate drinking, and if you are only drinking lightly, just two alcohol-free days will work wonders. Government safe-drinking guidelines recommend five days a week of no more than one or two small drinks, and two days per week without alcohol. For those who are worried their drinking might be getting out of hand, two weeks or even two days without any alcohol of any sort will be a great way of finding out if you can control your drinking. If you can't manage two weeks on the wagon, that's worrying, but if you can't go for two days, then you know something is seriously wrong.

Even when you are having a social drink on a night out, Five:Two has an answer that will also keep you healthy. For every five units of alcohol you consume, drink two large glasses of water or soft drink. Remember, a unit of alcohol is about half a glass of wine; or a single of spirits; or a third of a pint of beer.

> 1 glass of wine = 2 units
> 1 tot of whisky = 1 unit
> 1 pint of beer = 3 units

So for every couple of glasses of wine you drink, stop and drink a big glass of water – which is very European and therefore cool! For every pint and a half of beer you drink, you will need to drink a large glass of water. The sheer volumes of liquid involved here will be sure to slow down your consumption rate. On a big night out it is all too easy to drink as many units as government guidelines recommend for an entire week.

> **Max. Units Per Week**
> **For men = 21 units** (7 pints of beer)
> **For women = 14 units** (7 glasses of wine)

But by using Five:Two you can at least compensate by cutting your night's drinking with soft drinks and then balancing your overall intake by drinking less the rest of the week. So if you have a heavy night or even two, then no drinking for five days.

Not only does Five:Two fit in with healthy-living guidelines, it's also extremely simple. Here are the ratios you should use to put your drinking back in balance:

- **Five** units of alcohol: **two** large glasses water or soft drink
- **Five** days light-to-moderate drinking: **two** days without alcohol
- **Five** months of moderate drinking: **two** weeks on the wagon
- **Two** heavy evenings: **five** days completely teetotal

The formula for clubbing slow-down

Everybody loves a night out, and so we should. A change of environment; socializing with friends; raised heart rate from dancing – all these are fun and fit. What's not so great could be: legal and illegal highs; chaotic lifestyle and lack of sleep; poor decision making. When clubbing becomes a whole lifestyle, rather than just a simple night or two out, then things can start to get out of hand. According to doctors, people who sleep less than six hours a night are more likely to develop high blood pressure, cardiovascular disease and diabetes. Add in the increased risk of drug-taking, drinking too much, possible violence and sexual encounters, and a full-on clubbing experience doesn't sound like so much fun.

You will discover the perfect answer for getting your clubbing habits back where you can really enjoy them. The first type of balance is quite old-fashioned, but that's because it has been proved to work for a very long time. It's deceptively simple: save just two nights a week for clubbing, and spend the other five nights doing something else. So five alternative evenings; two nights clubbing. For most people that might mean Friday and Saturday, but it doesn't have to be. And you certainly don't have to spend the non-clubbing nights sat beside the fireside. Instead you can go to a dance class, or to a spin-cycle session, or to an acting club, or the cinema . . .

Another big rule to keep your clubbing under control is to allow yourself no more than five hours at a stretch, from the start of your evening. So if you are a 'pre-loader' who has a few drinks with mates before you hit the clubs, that means from then, not from the moment door security lets you into the club. If you start pre-loading at 7 p.m., then I'm afraid the ball will be over for you at midnight! Better to go and have a meal first, then start from around 9 or 10 p.m., which will take you to a normal 2 or 3 a.m.

Have you done things you regretted during a big night? Hmmm, maybe we all have. A simple rule is that for every five times you say 'yes' to something, then the next two times you must say 'no'. It can be a good game to play with yourself, or even with your whole party, and of course, if you actually *have* said 'no', then you won't end up wishing you had said 'no'. If you have a really bad track record on your nights out, you can switch to five 'no' and just two 'yes'.

Mark, the test pilot who has been having some issues stemming from clubbing, tried out the formula. He reported back via email: 'Stuck to two nights a week for the last few weeks. Joined the uni drama club for one of the not nights, and met someone. So went out with her for dinner one of the other not nights. Also got dosh coming in from shelf-stacking on not-nights. Went clubbing last night and had meal first. Very good, no stomach upset.' Mark usually has a takeaway kebab in the early hours at the end of a clubbing night, and he hadn't realized that was what caused his almost continuous bad stomach. So he started his night later, after a meal, and then said 'no' to a kebab – two good choices!

Cut your clubbing down to size

- **Five** nights of other activities: **two** nights of clubbing
- **Five** hours of clubbing: **two** hours resting or eating before
- **Five** 'yes' decisions: **two** 'no' decisions

The formula for social media and gaming management

When I first started my career as a journalist on a national newspaper in 1981, we used manual typewriters which made my fingers bleed. We didn't have either an office mainframe or personal computers, and there was no Google. We didn't even have mobile phones and there was no email. As a working journalist my life has been absolutely transformed by these things. I really do thank information technology on a daily basis for providing them. But I'm also glad that as a young journalist I didn't have to worry about managing my Facebook presence or my Twitter account, and I didn't have to bother about whether my media profile was trending sufficiently. If I wanted to sneak off for the day to watch the cricket, nobody could track me down by text or phone or email. A careless remark disappeared forever, and didn't find itself re-tweeted. An embarrassing moment at a family wedding never ended up on YouTube. If somebody was bullying me I could do something about it, straight away and face-to-face.

It's easy to forget that digital devices and social media are here to make life easier, not to make it more complicated and stressful. The digital world serves us, not the other way round. So if you are spending all day, every day checking your accounts and running your networking, it's time to bring it back under control. Or if an hour on your favourite game turns into the whole day and on into the night, you need to learn how to turn off as well as on.

Count how many devices and accounts you have. Including your phone, your media player, your laptop, your tablet, your TV, and then your various accounts – mail, online games, Twitter, Facebook etc – you can easily have more than a dozen. For the next five days you are only going to use two devices, and two accounts at a time. So if you are listening to your iPod at the same time as using your smart phone, that's it. You can't also be gaming, or have the TV on, or be using your PC or tablet.

And if you are texting someone and carrying on a chat-room conversation, you can't also have your Facebook open. You can choose which two you want, but you can't spread yourself across any more.

For two hours every day – best just before bed – all accounts are off. No checking email, no gaming, no taking texts or calls. Once you discover how much managing your media properly frees you up, you can consider having two days a week where you don't use media devices or accounts. This is especially helpful if you are unlucky enough to be attracting negative communications, as it gives you a chance to rest and relax. It usually breaks up the pattern of the communicator and often they will give up.

- **Five** or more devices and accounts? Use just **two** at a time
- **Two** hours a day without media
- **Two** days a week with a minimum of devices and accounts

The **Five:Two** Parenting Plan

It's one of the most important things any of us ever does in life. Most mums and dads also say it's what they are proudest of. Yet at the same time parenting is among the most difficult tasks you will ever face. And despite the millions of words written on the subject, each new parent has to learn how to do it from square one. No wonder parenting can seem like a minefield, or at times, even worse – a battlefield.

It shouldn't come as any surprise to learn that when Benjamin Spock, 'Dr Spock', published his book *Baby and Child Care* in 1946, it went straight to the top of the best-seller charts. Even today the book is still one of the biggest sellers of all time, outranked in its first fifty years only by the Bible. Whatever people think of his methods, one thing is certain: Dr Spock understood that people needed help with parenting.

Family influence

It wasn't that there hadn't been advice around before, in fact a lot of harassed mums found there was rather too much of it. With extended families, mothers, older sisters, grandmothers and parents-in-law all putting their oar in on how to bring up the new baby, the stay-at-home mums in the first half of the twentieth century probably felt just as pressurized as we do now. In some ways, though, life was more straightforward for mothers then. The wealthy classes largely delegated childcare to other people – nurses, nannies and schools – just as they had done for centuries. Everybody else assumed that the mother would take all responsibility for the children, usually giving up whatever they had been doing before the first child arrived.

Two world wars not only gave women the vote, they also showed that women could achieve just as much in the workplace as men. So by the time our own mothers and grandmothers were being born, there were a lot of questions being asked about what was the best approach to parenting, not just for the child, but for mum and dad as well.

Parenting choices

Today parents have a sometimes bewildering array of alternatives. Should dad take paternity leave? Should mum and dad look into the new options of shared leave over the first few years of the child's life? This is something that is already common in many European countries. Or what about opting for professional childcare? It can be expensive, but in theory it would leave you both free to continue your careers. Or how about establishing a good network of care amongst your extended family and in your close community? That can be an ideal answer if you are lucky enough to have it available.

And it's more than just a question of childcare. You have to decide what sort of parents you are going to be. Some parents change their whole lives when the children come along, and make parenting their main priority. Other parents like to keep a bit of their own identity and perhaps hope their children will grow up quite independent. The good news is that there is now awareness of more than one way of good parenting. And there is a lot more help and support for you in whatever choice you make.

Your choice

The less-good news is that, no matter how many workplace crèches and understanding bosses there may be out there to support whatever parenting choices you make, you do have to make some choices and no one else can do it for you.

You don't have to stick with your initial choices. I've known so many mums over the years determined to keep going with their careers, but once maternity leave was up they realized that being a mum was more important to them personally than being a company director. And I've also known a great many mums who've been brilliantly well organized and back at their desks before anyone has noticed they've gone.

Our test pilot Mary, now sixty-six, a Whitehall civil servant, has kept her high-flying career going through three children and as many government crises. She and her husband were among the first to make the decision that he would become a stay-at-home dad, which seemed to suit the whole family.

Choosing to have it all

At first Mary and her husband tried to have it all, as a great many of her generation of mums did. With feminists like Shirley Conran (whose book, *Superwoman,* was published in 1975) telling women that life was 'too short to stuff a mushroom' it was taken for granted that every woman wanted to be superwoman and to 'have it all'.

Nearly forty years later, the debate has changed from how to have it all to if it is actually possible, and whether women really want that anyway. Are women even being pushed into being working mothers because of the extra income they bring to the family? It is worth remembering that only fifty years ago it was uncommon for families to have a second car, or to take foreign holidays, let alone two foreign holidays a year. The fact that so many families can afford this now is largely due to having two full-time earners.

The Five:Two Parenting Formulas

Are you even having trouble becoming a parent in the first place? It's often forgotten that the first steps to successful parenting happen while the baby is still just a twinkle in mum and dad's eye. The special pre-conception formula can help you get pregnant when you want to and enjoy a smooth pregnancy. For a whole range of questions, issues and sometimes problems you face as a parent, the formulas will give you a framework to find the solution that is right for you.

Wherever you find yourself on the spectrum of parenting, Five:Two is here to help. Does 'having it all' just seem to mean 'having all the problems'? Our techniques can help you rebalance all the different claims on your time. You will discover how to focus on your true priorities at the same time as keeping other aspects of your life ticking over comfortably.

The Pre-conception and pregnancy formula

Surprisingly, one of the best things you can do for your child happens before you are even pregnant. There is so much research showing that healthy parents-to-be (both mum and dad) find it easier to get pregnant, and also have healthier babies, that the government is now advising parents to start thinking about this from at least three months before trying to start a baby.

Be positive about pregnancy health

The kind of changes you should make to your lifestyle to give you the best chance of quick, healthy and happy parenthood can sound quite strict, even frightening. But even though it sounds daunting, it has a very important plus. Everything you are doing for your baby, you are also doing for yourself. Remember that what is good for baby is good for you too. If you've always needed that extra little bit of motivation to give up smoking or to lose weight, your planned pregnancy will provide it.

The benefits will be immediate for your baby and they will also last you the rest of your life. Mary agrees with this: 'I'd always been a smoker and a red wine fan until my first pregnancy, when I gave up both. Now my three boys are grown-up and leaving home, and I'm still enjoying the benefits of being a non-smoker and drinking at a healthier level.'

Five:Two identifies five things that you need to be careful about before and during pregnancy, and two things to enjoy wholeheartedly.

Five things to be careful about

1. Vitamins and nutrition

One of the most obvious links between mum's nutrition and the baby's development is the birth of babies suffering from spina bifida. The first real research into this link was begun by Professor Richard Smithells in Liverpool in 1959, and thanks to this work, we now know the importance of having the right levels of a B-vitamin called folic acid. Today, seventy per cent fewer babies are born with spina bifida, due to correct vitamin supplementation for mothers-to-be. More research is showing that the importance of healthy eating goes even further than this. Foresight, the association for promoting pre-conception care, recommends a healthy diet with five helpings of fruit and vegetables; two helpings of protein (fish, meat etc.); and four helpings of grains (rice, porridge etc.) every day.

2. Overweight

It's unwise to go on a diet while you are pregnant, but preparing for pregnancy could be just the motivation you need to shift a few stubborn pounds. Women who are very overweight (BMI of thirty or more) can have problems getting pregnant. Pregnancy and birth can also be difficult. There is a higher chance of miscarriage, high blood pressure and a related condition called pre-eclampsia. Babies are slightly more likely to be born with problems and research has shown they are more likely to grow up to be overweight themselves.

3. Smoking

We all know the risks to our own health from smoking, but that goes double for our babies. The babies of smokers are born smaller than other babies and are more likely to be born prematurely, or to be stillborn. They are more likely to die as babies from sudden infant death (SID) and as they grow up they are more likely to develop asthma and other serious illnesses. If you manage to give up smoking, the benefits will be wonderful, not just for your baby but also for you. The pregnancy and birth are much more likely to go smoothly – and the general health improvement will last the rest of your life.

4. Drink and drugs

Alcohol, and drugs, can be very damaging to the formation of the baby and later to pregnancy and birth. Drinking before and during pregnancy has been associated with: miscarriage (over 9,000 women are admitted to hospital every year for miscarriages caused by alcohol: NHS Information Centre Hospital Admission data); low birth weight; heart defects; learning and behavioural disorders. The most severe of the alcohol-related conditions (which is normally due to heavy drinking in pregnancy) is Fetal Alcohol Syndrome (FAS). It causes: facial deformities; problems with physical and emotional development; poor memory or a short attention span.

The UK Chief Medical Officer's advice is: 'Women who are pregnant or trying to conceive should avoid alcohol altogether.' If you can't manage that, at the very least avoid alcohol while planning to become pregnant and in the first three months of pregnancy, because there may be an increased risk of miscarriage.

5. Diabetes

Being diabetic causes a number of risks during pregnancy and birth, but many women aren't aware they are diabetic. It is a good idea to have a general health check before you become pregnant, and especially a check for diabetes, blood pressure and healthy weight. If you discover you have diabetes, there's every chance of reversing it before you start your family.

Two things to enjoy

1. Taking care of yourself

All the health warnings surrounding parenthood can be seriously worrying! Some parents are so keen to do the right thing that they can start becoming obsessed with each new health warning and piece of research. The main thing to remember is that what's good for baby, is basically exactly the same as what is good for you. And this is one time in your life when nobody will criticize you for putting yourself first. So enjoy taking time to concentrate on your own health and well-being for a change – happy parents make happy babies!

2. Getting the baby buzz

Don't let your natural worries override the sense of joy everyone feels when there's a birth coming. Let yourselves have some treats. Let your friends have a baby shower for you. Check out the supermarket for all sorts of exciting – but non-alcoholic – health drinks that are now available. Buy a juicer. Even if you won't be drinking alcohol for months, you can still have fun!

The Childcare Formula

Childcare has become one of the hottest political issues around. Who should provide it? How much should it cost? Who should pay for it? How much should there be? Politicians and media commentators are constantly coming up with the answers to these questions. But we may not agree. When it comes down to it, the best person to answer the question is the parent – and the answer is going to be different for every parent. Take time before your baby is born to think very carefully about childcare – not just while your child is still a baby, but when he or she is growing up. Here's how to divide the different stages of your child's needs:

Get Me Everybody The pre-nursery stage when your baby needs you the whole time, both five Chunks and two Chunks of your attention.

Hands Full The toddler and nursery stage, when your child needs five Chunks but not the other two Chunks of your day.

Hands Half Full When your child is in full-time education and you can have five Chunks of life while your child is at school and then spend two Chunks of time for your child.

The 'Get Me Everybody' stage speaks for itself – you are going to need lots of help from family, friends and your workplace. At this stage there is little choice but to have your child as your main priority. Whatever your future plans, you will probably find it less stressful just to accept this.

The 'Hands Full' stage is the one with the hardest choices. Your child is off to nursery, so she doesn't need you to be physically there full-time. But does she need you at the gate? Or do you have someone you love and trust to help you? This is a good time to create your informal Care-Share network of family and friends.

Here's how the Care-Share works: it consists of five trusted people who would be happy to help in an occasional emergency; and two very close people – in practice grandparents or other family members – who would enjoy helping out more often. Your two close people might be providing a couple of afternoons a week of after-nursery childcare on a very regular basis. Your five other people would be there at the end of the phone in case something unexpected happens, and obviously would only need to be available for one in five emergencies. In return you would volunteer to help them out in the same way. This system can help provide back-up cover right through a child's life.

The 'Hands Half Full' stage may have slightly fewer direct time challenges, but it is far from straightforward. Many parents make the mistake of packing their children off to school with a sigh of relief that it's now up to the teachers. Even where schools offer breakfast clubs and homework clubs, your child will still only be in school supervision for a maximum of ten hours. With most schools it will be more like eight, or even slightly less if children are allowed off premises at lunchtime. What is going to happen to your child for the rest of the day and night? No matter how old your child, it is really important to know the answer to this question. Here's how to do it with five dos and two don'ts:

✓ Do take responsibility for your child, even if he or she is somewhere else

✓ Do be self-reliant, rather than depending on teachers or nurseries to do it all for you

✓ Do know where your child is, who she's with and a phone number, all the time

✓ Do plan ahead, especially for changes in routine

✓ Do think of every option, find out how other people have solved childcare issues

✗ Don't moan, it makes your child feel unloved

✗ Don't blame other people if things go wrong, the buck stops with mum or dad

The formula for education

They say schooldays are the best days of your life – but how about your children's schooldays being the best days of your own adult life? Take a positive approach and this can be a really happy time for the whole family. In Five:Two terms, your child may only need two Chunks of your time once he or she is at school full time. When it comes to your mental energy, though, you're likely still to be devoting a good five Chunks to your youngster – though they may be convinced they don't need it.

Choosing schools

The longer you plan ahead when it comes to choosing schools, the better your chances of getting a place at the right school for your child. It's unfortunate but true that you have to learn how to play the system. So make friends with parents of older children who've already been through it. Get active within the local school network. Visit online chat rooms and networks which have lots of information and useful leads. Remember to involve your child in the decision. He or she will certainly have an opinion, and it should be listened to – after all, they're the ones who will end up spending their days there, not you!

Any school can be the right school

Of course school is important, but ultimately it isn't as important to your child as you are. Teachers are great, but parents are better. You know your child better than anybody, and your child trusts you more than anyone else.

Maybe the school is a little weak in one area or another – you can do something about it. You can help your child directly by providing a good learning environment at home. Don't worry if it's not your specialist subject. You and your child can do the internet trawl together. Even more, you can get involved with the school. You don't have to go as far as being a parent governor, but you can volunteer with special projects and homework groups.

Five:Two your priorities

Remember the Chunks in Part One? A Chunk doesn't just have to be about time. A Chunk can be a cuddle or a conversation or having a good think. So even though you may only be able to spend two Chunks of time with your child each day, you can still give them five hugs, five interesting discussions, five listening sessions – and you'll probably be thinking about them even more than five Chunks!

Here are some balancing frameworks for this exciting stage in your child's life:

Communicating Five chats about anything; two chats on a subject you choose. Five listening moments; two times where you do the talking

Sharing Five Chunks on the computer together; two Chunks for your child in private. Five Chunks of your child playing with her friends; two Chunks where she is with you and the family

Rules Five times when you lay down the law; two times when he thinks he's got away with it

The formula for adolescence

Just when you have got childcare finally sorted out, and the right school, and you think you can finally relax, is the moment adolescence hits, and everything seems to be back at square one. Now more than ever, the Five:Two balance is going to help get things onto an even keel. Because, as every parent discovers, getting things into proportion is vital for steering your children into happy adulthood.

Five of love, two of tough

You can't be too hard on your teenagers, because they will just kick back even more. At the same time, there must be some ground rules, if only for your child's protection. The shorthand for this is simple: five of love, two of tough. You can provide your teenager with a home background that is basically loving and supportive, that will understand when things go wrong – that's the five of love. Your teenager also needs to know that there are a few really serious rules which they will get into big trouble at home for breaking – that's the two of tough.

The two of tough will vary from family to family. For me they come into two very simple categories. There is a tough rule against things that are dangerous to the teenager, like drug use or going into dangerous social situations (gangs etc.). The other tough rule is against things that are dangerous or anti-social to other people, like drink–driving or breaking the law. Most other situations can be covered from the five of love basis – that is by talking and working things through together as a family that basically loves each other.

The respect agenda

It's going to be rocky, and there may be times when you will resort to other sections of this book. You may even want to get your adolescent to read the section on Partying and Social Media. With all the tools provided here, you will be able to find ways of smoothing most stuff out, and simply coping with the rest of it. If you and your teenager can maintain a mutual respect and consideration for each other, things will go fine. You can start the respect agenda yourself by being sensitive and backing off a bit. Continue to involve your child in your family discussions. Calmly let him or her know how you feel about situations, and why certain things they do are upsetting you. At the same time, expect your teenager to continue to respect you. In Five:Two terms, you are showing five Chunks of consideration for your teenager, and you are looking for two Chunks of mutual respect. And one day, you will be rewarded by receiving a hefty five Chunks of love and respect from your grown-up child.

The **Five:Two**
Well-Being Plan

Do you remember being eleven or twelve years old and waking up in the morning on the first day of the school summer holidays? I hope you do, because with the Well-Being Plan you are going to recapture that wonderful feeling that you've probably forgotten about for years. Life used to be so full of possibilities. There were no worries, nothing hanging over you. And everything was such fun. Just going down to the supermarket was fascinating, and you could imagine all sorts of things. And there were big adventures too, like going to the beach for the day.

So what happened to that holiday feeling, that amazingly positive outlook? Life happened, of course, and you can't go on thinking like a child for ever. Yet surely it should be possible to become an adult without losing all of that sense of joy that we love so much in our children? Why does popping out to the supermarket no longer seem like a mini-adventure? Why has going for a day out on the beach become such a complex chore that we can't possibly fit it in? Most of us would identify stress as the chief reason why even what should be fun times, all

166

become just part of the daily grind. The UK charity, the Mental Health Foundation, agrees. Their research shows that every day about 250,000 people in the UK miss work because of stress. They also believe that seventy-five per cent of illness is stress related.

> 'Happiness is when what you think, what you say, and what you do are in harmony'
> MAHATMA GANDHI

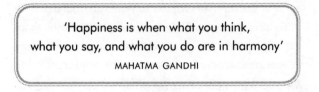

So what exactly is stress?

Stress is fashionable! During the Second World War, stress didn't exist. A few years ago I wrote a book about the sinking of a children's evacuation ship, the SS *Benares*, which was torpedoed by a German submarine as it crossed the North Atlantic. Nearly all the children died, but about twenty survived, and I interviewed those who were still living. I admired them all tremendously, and learnt so much from their survivor's attitude. One of them told me: 'When we were rescued we ended up back in Glasgow. They gave us clothes and stuff and we were waiting in a hall for our parents to come and fetch us. This bigwig came in with a uniform and I thought he was going to congratulate us on surviving, but he just said, "Buck up all of you." There was no thought of counselling or anything like that, which there would be now. You were just told: "There's a war on.'"

Does that mean stress is just a luxury that we indulge in because there's nothing else going on? Not quite. The bigwig's response was clearly not helpful to a young child, whether there was a war on or not. And some of the survivors I spoke to were still troubled, sixty years after the event. These people had been through an experience that was genuinely stressful. Yet how many people are diagnosed with 'stress' today, who aren't going through a genuinely stressful situation?

Does stress really exist?

Yes, stress does exist, but also no, it doesn't. The first thing to understand is that there is a big difference between actually *being* stressed – because you are genuinely in a very stressful situation – and *feeling* stressed. Many people face a lot of really awful stress in their lives, yet they don't feel stressed. Other people, whose lives might seem pretty comfortable to someone else, constantly complain of feeling stressed.

I interviewed a wonderful man recently who had been a Colour Sergeant in the Royal Marine Commandos, serving in a particularly nasty spot in the Helmand province of Afghanistan. By any standards, that is a genuinely stressful situation. Yet, under this horrible stress, he was able to start a dog rescue charity,

Nowzad, which as I write this book, has rehomed more than 600 dogs rescued in war theatres by servicemen. On the other hand, various friends, on hearing about this book, have responded by telling me how stressed they are. Even though they aren't actually in a stressful situation, they *feel* stressed.

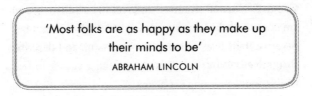

'Most folks are as happy as they make up
their minds to be'

ABRAHAM LINCOLN

Four stress types

The sad thing is that people who *feel* stressed, even though they aren't in a genuinely stressful situation, can be much more miserable and unwell than people who are plunged into the midst of stressful events. When it comes to stress and personality, there are four ways it can go:

Group A: Stressful situation and feel stressed This happens where people are suddenly put in frightening situations and find that they can't cope. This often gives rise to what is called Post Traumatic Stress Disorder (PTSD).

Group B: Stressful situation and feel OK Many people, in exactly the same situation as Group A, are able to cope and function well, and even after the event they do not develop PTSD. As yet there is no conclusive answer as to why there is this difference, and there needs to be a lot more research.

Group C: Normal situation and feel stressed This group are not in acutely dangerous or frightening situations, but perceive their lives as being very stressful, and describe themselves as stressed. This feeling can give rise to real health and well-being problems.

Group D: Normal situation and feel OK Luckily most of us fall into this group, plodding on as normal. Our lives are actually very similar to those in Group C, but we don't think of them as being particularly stressful, and we don't feel particularly stressed.

Solutions for all

All the different stress personality groups can be helped out of their stress. It's really important for Group A – the endangered stressed – to get help from professionals, and fortunately the position is now much better than it was in the Second World War. Group B – endangered but coping – also need to think a little more about their situation so they can continue to cope long after the immediate source of stress is over. And again, it's important that they do so. Research has found that the Five:Two method of thinking about the situation, and revisiting it mentally, in a controlled way, works better at preventing PTSD than simply going on as though everything is fine. Groups A and B will need some face-to-face help with their revisiting technique.

If you are feeling stressed, you are probably quite convinced that you are in a situation every bit as stressful as those in Group A, but this might not really be the case. There may well be other reasons why you feel stressed, and that's what this book is here to help with. Some people definitely need to get in touch with health carers. However, many people in Group C, who *feel* stressed but don't have any very obvious sources of stress in their lives, can do a lot for themselves – especially once they learn how to balance their lives.

So let's start thinking about your feelings of stress. The picture below is a 'stress cloud'. It shows the really serious causes of stress in our lives. If you can identify one of these in your life – even from many years ago – that could well be why you are suffering from stress now. Reading this book will help, but you should also get face-to-face advice and treatment from a specialist.

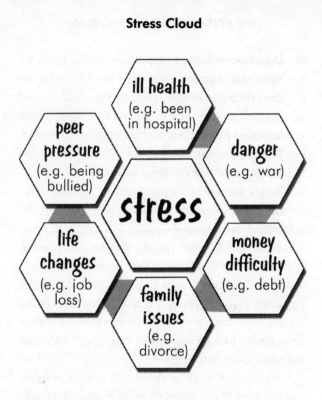

Feeling stressed – but not sure exactly why

The experiences highlighted in the Stress Cloud are what I call the 'big bad events'. If your husband has just left you, or you're in serious financial difficulty, or you are being nastily bullied, there are no ifs or buts. These things are awful. But how about if you can't really point to anything that bad in your life? Yet you feel stressed. These are the kind of statements you might identify with:

* Don't know what will happen
* Too much to do
* Can't sleep properly
* Worried about everything
* Irritable with people
* Nothing seems to go my way
* Afraid I can't manage things I have to do
* Family feels out of control
* Just wish I could have a piece of luck
* Nobody is on my side

Time to Five:Two for a new you

These are the feelings this book is here to help you with. You are going to learn to approach your negative feelings in a new way – two little bits at a time. We are going to discover what might be the source of your feelings, and then you can pick the right formula to help you rebalance your life.

For the next five days, please set aside two short sessions every day to have a proper think about your feelings and your life. Your sessions don't need to be very long, but they must be quiet and in private, so that you can concentrate. I set my alarm clock twenty minutes earlier and creep downstairs to have a cup of coffee and a little think.

The test pilots have started off by making a life staircase. This is a chart which shows how your feelings about life go up and down over the years. The steps are five-year periods of your life, from birth to seventy-five years old. All you have to do is rate how happy you felt in each period on a scale of –5 to +5, with –5 being absolutely miserable, and +5 being ecstatically happy. Zero is for neutral, don't know or can't remember – which is obviously where the first five years usually are.

Here's test pilot Mary's life staircase:

Mary's Life Staircase

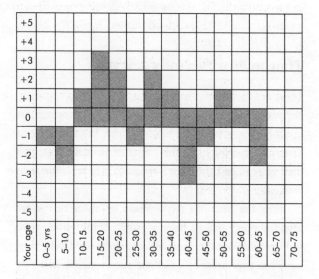

Just a quick glance shows Mary's life has been going up and down stairs like a game of snakes and ladders. No wonder she's feeling low, stressed and anxious. Now she needs to look at what happened in her life in the past to cause those peaks and troughs. Then she will be able to find out the things that really make her happy in life, and also what has been upsetting her well-being.

> 'The happiness of your life depends
> upon the quality of your thoughts'
> MARCUS AURELIUS

For a contrasting life staircase, I asked Rob, one of the 'air controllers', to fill in the life staircase:

Rob's Life Staircase

	0–5 yrs	5–10	10–15	15–20	20–25	25–30	30–35	35–40	40–45	45–50	50–55	55–60	60–65	65–70	70–75
+5															
+4				■		■	■								
+3			■	■	■										
+2		■	■		■	■									
+1		■	■	■	■	■	■	■							
0	■	■	■	■	■	■	■								
−1									■	■					
−2										■					
−3										■					
−4															
−5															

Your age

Rob talked me through his staircase: 'I don't remember that much about my early childhood, I guess it was just normal. But things really took off for me when I went away to a boarding school and started playing rugby. I loved it – and it loved me! Looking back, I think I partly got my place at uni because they were so big on rugby, and I captained the team. I got injured around the time I graduated, which was a shame, but a rugby contact helped me get a good job and I was so busy that although I missed the rugby, it didn't become a huge negative in my life. Then pretty soon afterwards I was married and our first child came along. I remember my early thirties as just being great!

'Things started to slide after the birth of our third child. It wasn't diagnosed at the time, but I think my wife must have been suffering from post-natal depression. I don't really know. But anyway, things never really picked up again after that. Eventually she started divorce proceedings and it got a bit nasty. There've been a lot of allegations flying round and the lawyers are always involved. I'm finding it really difficult to get the opportunity to spend time with my kids and that's just very hard. I have to admit I'm at the lowest point I've ever been.'

Now have a go at filling in your own staircase. Don't overthink it at first. Just quickly consider: plus or minus? Very plus or very minus? The time to think about it is when you have filled in your staircase and you can suddenly see your life on paper. It may be quite revealing.

Your Life Staircase

Your age	0–5 yrs	5–10	10–15	15–20	20–25	25–30	30–35	35–40	40–45	45–50	50–55	55–60	60–65	65–70	70–75
+5															
+4															
+3															
+2															
+1															
0															
−1															
−2															
−3															
−4															
−5															

FIVE:TWO FOR A NEW YOU

The Five:Two Well-Being Formulas

The formula for tired all the time

I expect any family doctor reading this is now groaning.
It must be the most common complaint doctors get in
their surgeries, and only occasionally is there an obvious
physical reason. Sometimes there don't seem to be
any psychological answers either. You don't feel really
depressed, it's just an all-round sigh situation. The answer
is actually much more simple than we might imagine.
I think the reason we get tired all the time is because we
aren't generating any new energy in ourselves.

Where might we generate new energy from? From
pleasure, from a little fun, through having a joyful
moment. We are not talking foreign holidays with every
changing season. All it takes is a couple of chuckles a day.
Remember how great it used to feel dancing round the
house? Or how energized you feel after a good laugh? Or
even singing in the shower? But then maybe some difficult
life event happened, and you just got out of the habit.

Put fun back in your life – on a daily basis!

This is one formula that has to be done every day: For
every five times you feel tired, or low, or too exhausted
to do the next thing, you are going to have two moments
of pure fun. Here's a list of little things – some silly – to
do or say that are just going to be for fun.

Power pleasure moments

- Do an email (it will be too long to text or tweet) of the shaggiest dog story you know and send it round your mates and colleagues
- Have a kiddy-style ice cream – they still make Fabs and 99s!
- Sing
- Enjoy a damn fine cup of coffee or a proper pot-made cup of tea
- Make up an idiotic nickname for yourself
- Find something to enjoy about the weather, no matter what it is
- Put on your favourite sweater
- Think of your favourite image or painting, and find it online or buy a postcard of it
- If you're female put on some lipstick; if you're male, hey why not!
- Dance
- Stroke a cat or dog or hamster (get its permission first!)
- Watch your favourite movie
- See one thing, any thing, that you think is lovely, whether it's the sky or a girl walking down the street

If you can get a moment or two like this into every day of your life, I guarantee you will stop feeling so tired.

The formula for loneliness

What with texts and tweets and Facebook and smart phones and tablets and all the zillions of ways we humans now have of being together, you would think loneliness would be a thing of the past. But nothing can make you feel lonelier than being 'trolled'. And if you have lost someone you love, no amount of action on the smart phone is going to make up for it. All the same it is perfectly possible to be alone without being lonely.

Psychologists divide personality into two types: extrovert and introvert – phrases we all tend to throw about. Most of us have friends who are typical extroverts – the life and soul of the party. Perhaps you're an extrovert yourself. But what few of us notice is the downside of being an extrovert, that when the party's over, you can feel very lonely. Whereas introverts, who maybe didn't appear to be enjoying the party so much at the time, have the pleasure of remembering it inwardly once it's over.

Balancing your personality type

Decide whether you are an extrovert or an introvert – most of us already have a pretty good idea of this. Now you have to balance your personality type.

Extroverts should balance their five outward-looking activities with two inward-looking, thinking activities.

Introverts should balance their five inward-looking activities with two outward-looking, social activities.

Balancing activities for extroverts

❖ Read a difficult book – the more thought-provoking the better

❖ Start writing a diary

❖ For a night out go to the cinema or theatre rather than clubbing

❖ Let a friend know something personal about yourself

❖ Swap a team sport like football for an individual sport like tennis or running

Balancing activities for introverts

❖ Join, join, join! Any kind of club that has regular meetings

❖ For every five times you say no to an opportunity, say yes twice, and aim to get the ratio up to five yes and two no

❖ Next time you are at a social or work gathering, introduce yourself to at least two people you don't know

❖ Phone two friends you haven't spoken to recently

❖ Have your coffee or lunch at the café rather than taking out

The formula for worried about worrying

Oddly enough it's often the best copers who are also the biggest worriers. People who believe they should be able to manage a certain situation, or put everything right that has gone wrong, then start feeling very responsible and pressurized if things get out of hand. After a while, the worrying becomes a habit. The Chunking techniques from Part One are very useful when it comes to breaking this vicious circle.

Here's how to do it: You have something difficult to deal with and you are worrying about it. Perhaps you are trying to cope with a stressful situation within the family, or maybe even a legal problem. Now you are going to Chunk your approach to this problem. Certainly you are going to think about the problem and deal with it, but you are also going to have times when you aren't directly doing anything about it and when you aren't thinking about it.

Chunks of worry, and also Chunks of not worrying

Of course you need to engage with your problem. You can't ignore it completely, especially if it involves legal meetings, paperwork etc. Allocate time and mental energy to these elements – but don't give all your time and energy to it. Do what needs to be done, and when that has been done, stop worrying until the next time something needs to be done. If you reply to a letter, there's nothing you can do until you get a response back to your reply. Wait until that moment comes before you start worrying again. If you are in a tough situation, you may have to spend five Chunks of your time and energy dealing with it, but make sure you have two Chunks of not worrying. A more minor problem might allow you to spend five Chunks of your mental energy not thinking about it, as long as you devote two Chunks to getting it sorted out.

An appointment to worry

There are lots of mind games you can play with yourself, like 'filing away' worried thoughts, to help you Chunk up your worries, and you can read about them in Part Three. But many of us get worried about whether we are worrying enough! Test pilot Mary emailed me: 'I'm trying to have not-worried Chunks, but I'm worried that if I do that I might forget something, or things might slide more if I'm not worrying about them . . .' So I've asked Mary to make herself 'an appointment to worry'. She's allowed to worry, not more than five Chunks, and she can write down in her diary the times she's allocated for that. Mary tried this for a few weeks and rang to say: 'That's really helping. I find I can look at my diary and see that I'm going to be doing the worrying all day on Thursday – weirdly I then relax and think "Oh I don't need to worry now, I'm worrying on Thursday." It does feel a bit peculiar though.'

I'm hoping that when 'worry appointments' come round, Mary may actually start feeling a little less worried even then – but I'm waiting for the next report.

The formula for bad nights

Comedian and author David Baddiel found a way round his chronic insomnia – he used his sleepless nights to write a best-selling novel about sleepless nights. So being a bad sleeper isn't all negative. It's hard to believe that when your nights are spent tossing and turning, and then when you do get to sleep, you end up having nightmares. Psychiatrists have identified that one of the major problems with insomnia is that it sets up a vicious circle, where the poor sufferer becomes so worried about not getting enough sleep, that they start losing sleep over it . . .

Now break that vicious circle

For five nights every week, begin this wind-down to sleep two hours before you go to bed:

❖ Have a warm (not over-hot) bath or shower and change out of day clothes
❖ Eat a meal including starchy carbohydrates (bread, pasta, rice, potatoes) and lettuce – lettuce actually contains a substance which causes sleepiness!)
❖ Don't drink alcohol or caffeine
❖ Switch off all media devices including computer, tablet, mobile phone
❖ Don't take or make phone calls or tweet or text
❖ Listen to gentle music, or watch dull television or read a book
❖ Don't have any media devices in the bedroom
❖ Change your sheets often
❖ When in bed have a cuddle with your partner
❖ When you have switched the light out you need to stay in control of your thoughts by meditating, or even telling yourself little stories (use the tips in Part Three)

The other two nights, don't bother with any of these good sleep habits. It is quite likely that at first you are not going to sleep well for the two 'not bothering' nights. The only thing you have to do on those two nights is accept your wakefulness. Be comfortable that it is only this one or two nights. Use that wakeful time to catch up on some reading – or write a diary. Allow yourself to rest and relax. Try some meditation. Remind yourself that rest is every bit as helpful to you as sleep. Most people who follow this pattern gradually find that their sleep improves to the point where they sleep pretty much as well on the good sleep habit nights as on the not bothering nights.

'Happiness is not something ready made.
It comes from your own actions'
DALAI LAMA

PART THREE
Your **Five:Two**
Tool Kit

Introducing the Tools You Need

The goal-setting technique in Part One, combined with your chosen plan (or plans) from Part Two will set the path for you to go on a new life journey. And just to make things easier along the way, this part of the book gives you a full set of tools to use when you are working on your plan.

Mind Games

I believe that most of the things we tussle with in life can be resolved by using Five:Two techniques. The plans in this book are very practical and straightforward. They concentrate on positive goals, and things you can do now to improve or change a situation that is bothering you. In addition, you can make it even easier by learning to adjust your frame of mind. The tips here are largely drawn from Cognitive Behaviour Therapy (CBT), a way of thinking which psychologists have developed to help people cope when they feel stressed, worried or unhappy. These simple 'mind games' can ultimately change your outlook on life with a few basic techniques for taking control of your mindset. Give them a try to help you while you follow your Five:Two plan – and afterwards.

Meditation

Forget chanting and ringing bells, meditation isn't at all mystic. The word 'meditation' relates to letting your conscious day-to-day mind go, so that you can access what is going on underneath, what some people call the subconscious mind. The subconscious is really just the stuff that goes on all the time in the back of your mind without you being really aware of it. It's a bit like all that software that runs in the background on your computer that you only notice is running when you come to shut your computer down. And that's pretty much what meditation is – a way of shutting down all the applications, so that you can see what's running in the background.

Accessing your subconscious

Becoming aware of what's going on in your subconscious mind is a wonderfully liberating thing to do. Our subconscious is both very powerful, and extremely good at taking care of business. You know if you need to wake up in the morning and you wake just before the alarm clock? That's your subconscious clock, which ticks the whole time. Or if you have been chewing over a thorny problem, then wake up the next day knowing the solution, again that's the subconscious.

So being able to access our subconscious mind whenever we need to, rather than having its effects just popping up randomly, is very helpful. Sometimes the subconscious is grappling with something we'd rather not think about, and that also needs to be addressed as it can be part of Post Traumatic Stress Disorder (PTSD). For many reasons then, we sometimes want to have a look at those background programmes.

Shutting down

Look up towards the ceiling and gently close your eyes as you count to three. Relax. Think about yourself relaxing. Feel your muscles relax, every one from your forehead down to your toes. You can think: 'I'm calm and safe' if you want. Now imagine you are walking down towards one of your favourite places. Perhaps you are walking down some steps onto the beach. Or you are walking down the hill towards a picnic spot you like. Or you are walking down a path to a seat in a forest clearing. Wherever you end up should be completely empty of people. Spend some time in this place. If you have a problem or something you particularly want to think about, now is the time to do it. Or if you have just been tired and need a rest, you can simply lie back and soak up the lovely atmosphere of your special place.

It is quite likely you will doze off for a few minutes. When you wake up, or when you want to finish your meditation, allow yourself to drift gently back to the world. Remind yourself that you are calm and safe, and then open your eyes.

Solutions

Meditators find this technique a powerful tool for solving difficult issues. In my experience you don't necessarily come up with the answer straight away, but somehow the solution suddenly becomes obvious, thanks to your subconscious. Often I find that if I have a nap during a meditation I wake up re-energized with a strong idea of what to do next.

Relaxation

Because meditation requires a state of relaxation, many people confuse the two, but relaxation isn't about problem solving or thought in the way that meditation is. Relaxation is about letting go completely, with both your conscious and your subconscious mind. It is the most simple form of downtime which we all need. When people meditate they usually do so with an objective in mind, but the whole idea of relaxation is to get away from objectives for a while.

The treats that relax

One of the best ways of relaxing is to have a favourite treat. It doesn't need to be a big treat, in fact it seems to work better if it is a small treat that won't make you feel guilty. The treats that work for me are: a cup of good fresh coffee; a country walk; half an hour sitting in the sun in the back garden. What makes them relaxing is that nothing disturbs them, and I can enjoy them without thinking about anything else. It doesn't even have to be that sunny to sit out – as long as it's not actually raining.

Relax Lucky Dip

Think about your favourite relaxing treats and make a list of them. Write each one down on a scrap of paper and fold them up. Put them all in a container. When you know you need to have a relaxing moment, go to the Relax Lucky Dip and pull yourself out a treat.

Positive thinking

This is another useful mind game that, like meditation, accesses the subconscious. Like everything associated with the subconscious, it is very powerful. However, this mind game is quite hard to play. It involves taking out all the negative phrases from your thinking. For example, imagine you want to give up smoking. You might think to yourself: 'I'm not going to smoke any more.' Although that's a good thing to want, you are expressing it as a negative: 'I'm *not* . . .'

Now try to think of some ways of saying this without using a negative word. It's quite tricky. Many people come up with the phrase: 'I have smoked my final cigarette' as a way of expressing positively their will to quit.

Negative expressions every day

We all use negative expressions a surprising amount in day-to-day life. How often do you say or think 'I can't . . .' during the day? Try to notice all those negative phrases and replace them with positive ones.

It can be quite an eye-opener to see that our general attitude is often quite negative. Often we think: 'Oh, I don't want to . . .' Now how about thinking what you *do* want. Put positives first: 'I will get through a good chunk of work today, and then I can go late-night shopping.' That's two positives: 'will' and 'can'. Just changing the way you express things in your mind gradually builds up into a massively more positive outlook on your whole life. So replace 'not' and 'don't' and 'can't' with 'will' and 'can' and 'do'.

Banking

This is one of my favourite mind games, and I like to think I invented it, but probably it's just been absorbed by my subconscious from somewhere else. The idea of banking is just like the piggy bank you might have had as a child, except that instead of putting money in it, you are going to put happiness into it. So a particularly happy moment gets put into the bank. The bank can be a real bank – like a diary or a ledger that you write your happy moment into, just like depositing a cheque. I have a book that I write my happy moments into – and recently had to start a new one. It doesn't matter what the happy moment is. It could be something you or a family member has achieved. Or it could be a lovely time you had with friends or family. Or it could just be a fun, happy feeling you had for no apparent reason.

I concentrate on things that were happy and that I enjoyed rather unexpectedly. Occasionally I have to go on a particular work assignment that I dread, but sometimes they actually turn out to be great fun and I come back having had a happy time. Those moments are just right for putting into the bank.

Like every bank, you can make withdrawals as well as deposits. So if you are feeling down, you can go to your happiness bank and take one of the happy moments out and re-experience it. And even better, you can withdraw as often as you want, and your happiness account never gets smaller. Try to make sure you keep paying in new happy moments.

Filing

This is more or less the opposite of banking, and I know I didn't invent this mind game, as it has been used for a long time by psychologists and by hypnotherapists to help people deal with unpleasant or negative situations. I find it is particularly helpful if there is something stressful that I am worrying about all the time, even though I only need to engage with the situation once in a while. Basically what you are doing in this mind game is telling your subconscious to put its worries away in the file, either for the time being, or permanently.

Here's the filing technique: Perhaps you have an ongoing stressful situation. It could be something like a redundancy process, where your employer will be holding a series of meetings and consultations where they will decide who will be made redundant and how much payment they will receive. This is obviously a horrible time for everyone concerned. You know you are going to have to attend at least a couple of meetings that may be unpleasant. So you are worried about it. In fact you worry about it all the time, and you are losing sleep about it. In reality though, you only need to worry about these meetings when you are about to have them – the point at which you need to make any preparations, and then actually have the meeting. Worrying the rest of the time isn't helpful.

So get yourself into a meditation situation. When you are down in that nice, happy place, imagine a door. Open the door and find yourself in a library. There are a number of book stacks on your left and right. On the left hand side you find a book about your redundancy worry. You glance through it and then close it firmly. On your right-hand side there is a shelf marked 'filed'. You put the book onto the 'filed' shelf and leave it there, walking out of the library with the book closed and filed. By doing this you are telling your subconscious that it can let go of its worry, because it is on the shelf.

If you're worrying situation is ongoing, you can make a date in your mind when you need to take the book back down before putting it away again. But you don't need to think about it before that date arrives.

Into the Shredder

If the stressful or upsetting event is over, you can have a more final way of dealing with your worries or anxiety. Perhaps you've just been through a really difficult break-up. It's all over now, but somehow your mind won't let go of it and you find yourself dwelling on it all the time.

Go into the library of your subconscious again. This time you will notice that at the end of the corridor of book stacks there is a heavy duty shredder machine. Look on the left book shelf and pull down the book about your ended relationship. Don't even bother to open it. Just take it straight down to the end of the corridor and put it through the shredder. You'll be surprised how successful this technique is.

Changing Sides

This interesting mind game is one that psychologists use a lot when they are teaching Cognitive Behaviour Therapy (CBT). Sometimes our anxieties in life stem from faulty thinking on our part – but it's not always easy to spot that.

Imagine a friend is walking down the opposite side of the high street. You're in too much of a rush to stop and say hello, but you give her a friendly wave, only to be met with nothing. Has your friend fallen out with you? Was it something you said? You are fretting all day until you manage to get your friend on the phone. That's when you hear that she didn't see you, or perhaps had just had some bad news and didn't want to talk. So it was nothing to do with you at all.

The other point of view

How about a workplace scenario, where your boss is being absolutely impossible to you. Irritable, demanding, distant. You start to get more and more worried. Has your standard of work slipped? Is your boss looking to replace you with someone else? Are you going to get the sack? It's not until several days have passed, and you've become really anxious, that you hear on the grapevine that your boss is about to be side-lined by a massive reorganization that will do away with her current role. So again, your boss's behaviour had nothing to do with you, and everything to do with her own problems.

If you are feeling worried or confused about your relationships with other people, whether it's in your personal life or elsewhere, use the changing sides technique to work out what's causing their behaviour.

Walk a mile in their moccasins

If the shop assistant is being rude and unhelpful, get into her shoes. Maybe she hasn't been in the job long and feels out of her depth. Maybe she genuinely hasn't got enough training or backing from management to help you with your query. She may be feeling very worried herself and is therefore being defensive.

Knowledge is powerful

Once you realize these possibilities, you can react accordingly. Based on your knowledge, you can reach out to the other person and this can lead to surprisingly good results, as well as reassuring your own anxieties.

Going Into Neutral

When things are getting really tough, this clever little tool can make a difference very quickly. Psychologists have found that one of the biggest problems encountered by people who are feeling down is that they enter a vicious circle. They are feeling a bit down, which is a bit worrying and a bit confusing, so they get slightly depressed about feeling down. Then, because they are depressed, they focus on that feeling and allow it to dominate; after all, you can't have a good time when you are depressed, can you? Pretty soon, someone who was only in a slightly low mood is genuinely depressed.

It is the same with any number of different unpleasant feelings. If you are anxious about some stressful event, it's only natural to start getting a bit worried about how anxious you feel, and then the whole thing builds up until you can't think of anything else.

Have the emotion without the emotion

The mind trick of 'going into neutral' aims to break this vicious circle. It is very simple. Don't be worried about being worried. Don't let yourself get depressed about being depressed. Don't feel sad about being sad. Accept the emotion you are feeling, and just go with the flow. Yes, I might be depressed or worried about something, and either I will eventually get on top of it, or it will sort itself out. But in the meantime I don't need to fret about it. Just because I'm going through a tough time doesn't mean I can't enjoy a movie. Psychologists call this 'having the emotion without the emotion'. Once you've got used to it, it's very liberating – if a slightly odd feeling at first.

Mood turn around

There are some fancy names for this technique, but it has actually been known about, and used for ever. It may not always have had psychological names like 'mindfulness' and so on, but basically it is the scientific version of: 'Cheer up, love, it may never happen.'

Even if 'it' has actually happened, you still have the power to turn your mood right around. Just think of a time when you were happy. Use your happiness bank, described above. Now imagine yourself feeling as you did then, think 'What if I was happy right now?' Then give yourself permission to feel like that.

Smiling is a two-way street

There are physical things you can do to help you achieve this. Just smile or laugh. You don't have to mean it. Sing a happy song. Scientists have discovered that the neural pathways involved in smiling and chuckling actually work in both directions. So when we are happy or pleased or amused, we smile. The surprising thing is that it goes the opposite way too. So if you smile and laugh quite a bit, eventually you will start feeling happier, even if you were quite down before you started smiling. This may be one of the reasons comedians are so popular.

Tuning-in

The science behind this involves a part of the brain called the amygdala, which is now known to play a vital role in our emotional reactions, our memory and our ability to learn. It is associated with what is known as 'emotional intelligence' which helps us communicate with our fellow human beings and is profoundly linked with creativity and the ability to have feelings. Some new research has shown that our amygdala is changing and developing all the time.

Scientists now believe that we may be able to tune into our amygdala in such a way that we can increase our ability to empathize with others and join in mutual creative processes. The research is in its early days, but there is some suggestion that by concentrating on creative experiences (like looking at a beautiful painting) or even just thinking happy thoughts, we can increase positive activity in the amygdala. Why not give it a try?

PART FOUR
Hot Off the Press

How Did Everyone Get On?

The test pilots report back

When I began writing and researching *Five:Two For a New You*, friends and family volunteered to be guinea pigs testing out the formulas, and they have been keeping in touch throughout. Now that we've all reached the end of the book, here are their final reports back in.

Stew

Stew did the Fitness Plan because he wanted to get back into shape again and was finding it hard now that he's got his own business. He used the goal-setting techniques in Part One to set a fitness goal. Here's his verdict:

'Yeah, I think this is definitely working. It's hard to tell because my goal – to compete in the triathlon – isn't until the spring, so I'm not there yet. But the big thing that's worked for me is that my little boy is getting stuck into it. He's been in a fun run with me and won a medal. Now he wants a proper bicycle. He thinks he's Bradley Wiggins. It's turned out great really, because I'm enjoying all this stuff with my son, and that's the best bit about it.'

Mary

Mary wanted to try all the different plans in this book. I persuaded her to start out with the Well-Being plan, where she also filled in her Life Staircase to get an idea of the happy and less happy times in her life so far. She emailed me:

'I read the plans the whole way through before I began doing anything. I know you were keen for me to do the Well-Being plan, so I started there, which probably was the right thing because it meant I filled in the staircase. That was a big eye-opener. It really made me think about the times I have been happiest, and why I was happy then. I loved school, and university, and if I'm honest I enjoyed my job, even though it was so high pressure.

'After thinking about all that, I started with the plans again. This time I looked at Work/Life Balance, Relationships and – which really surprised me – Parenting. I've realized that I'm giving too much time and emotional energy to the men in my life, three sons and a husband. So I'm working on that. I've told the boys – well, let's face it, they're young men now – that they must do more for themselves.

'I'm not sure I can report back any big achievements, except that now I actually know where to start. I'm setting a goal, and I'm going to use Five:Two properly this time. I'm really quite excited about it!'

Mark

Mark is the youngest of the test pilots, and he was still at university when we started researching the book. He was beginning to worry that his life was getting away from him a bit after a few hard words from his boss on a recent work placement. We had a coffee together for his report:

'Everything basically has changed. I've got a girlfriend, a degree and almost a full-time job. So I'm totally sorted. But I think that would probably have happened anyway without your Five:Two plan,' he said.

'Hang on, what about you telling me how you met your girlfriend?'

'Yes, well obviously that was because of that bit in the plan where you said to go to the theatre group instead of clubbing or staying in and gaming. And I met her at the theatre group.'

'And what about this almost-job?'

'I suppose I did start the shelf-stacking because of the plan, and it's the shelf-stacking that got me the management traineeship at the supermarket. But it would all have worked out OK in the end anyway.'

He's probably right. The advantage of being young is that life gives you plenty of chances to get over the occasional wrong path, but I still think that without Five:Two it would have taken him a lot longer.

Steph

Steph was the first to volunteer to test pilot *Five:Two For a New You*. It's typical of her enthusiasm and energy that she jumped right in. She emailed me:

'I love it all! I read the whole thing and I like that it's punchy and totally accessible.'

For Steph the big plus was that it is something she can fit into her busy life quite easily. She particularly liked using the 'Chunking' techniques to rebalance the various elements of her life without having to make huge changes. She says: 'I'm going to go on with Chunking and Five:Two ideas even though we've finished the research.'

Me

I first came across some of the principles behind Five:Two several years ago when I was doing a course on Cognitive Behaviour Therapy. CBT, as it's known, has received the highest endorsement and it is now available free by prescription at some medical practices. It's a form of psychological counselling which focuses on understanding the world around you and how you interact with it. It's also very solution-oriented, so it tends to be positive and down to earth.

When I started to research and write this book I knew immediately that much of what I had learnt about CBT would be relevant. CBT has a lot of advice about achieving balance and a sense of proportion in your life. Five:Two is all about balance and proportion. The idea of having a balance between five of one thing and two of another feels instinctively right. So when I started planning this book it gave me a chance to write about ideas that I believed in, and had already been using for quite a while.

Five:Two For a New You gave me the framework to put those ideas down in writing – and to work through my thinking in detail. I found writing the book really enjoyable. Plus, I was putting the principle into practice the whole time. As you know, my main goal was to write this book, which I'm glad to say, has been achieved.

My other goal was to run a 26.2 mile full marathon in aid of charity. I did that last weekend and I did manage to finish. My time wasn't great, just on the four hours fifty minutes mark, and yes I was Five:Two-ing those lamp posts again!

The air controllers report back

When I recruited my 'test pilots' to test out the ideas in this book, I wanted to be as scientific as possible, so I also asked two friends to act as a 'control' group. They wouldn't use Five:Two so that we could compare how they got on without it versus those who were using it.

Rob

Rob had originally volunteered to be a test pilot, but agreed to be a controller at least while the research was going on. He acted as a control on filling in the Life Staircase. He caught up with me the other day:

'I'm feeling much better than when I was helping with *Five:Two For a New You*, mainly because the aftermath of my divorce has settled down a bit. I'm getting much better access to the kids, partly because I'm not working abroad so much now, which makes it easier to arrange the access days.

'But – and it's a big but – I feel a huge cheat. What happened was that filling in the life staircase, made me have a big think about things.

'I looked at when I was really happy in my life, and it was when the children came along. I'd been a bit low after having to give up rugby, but the kids more than made up for it. Then I realized I was stupid to be putting work, having to work abroad, as a higher priority than seeing them. So I went and talked to my boss and we changed my role so that I wouldn't have to go abroad so much. So, in a way, I have done Five:Two and I haven't been a proper control. Sorry.'

Melanie

Melanie was my ideal 'air controller' for the research, because she didn't agree with the principles of Five:Two and felt that her life was going really well in every way. She emailed me:

Glad to hear you've finished the book, it sounds like you had fun writing it. I've been in the wars a bit lately because I tore my ACL (anterior cruciate ligament) doing some hard-core training in the gym. It's been a real pain, in every way! I've had it operated on and I was on crutches for a few weeks. Doing the rehab fine, but I've had to be off work for a while and got a bit out of touch.

Have to admit the physio said I'd probably been fraying the ligament for quite a while, she thought I might have been overdoing the high-impact stuff.

I went to see Mel to say get well soon and because she seemed slightly depressed in her mail – who wouldn't be! We had an interesting chat about the knock-on effects of her injury. Her main social circle of friends are connected with work and going out together after work. When she was off work, Mel missed out on that. She was also quite surprised by how excluded she felt from her social circle while she was on crutches. 'It was like it was all just too much trouble – getting me into the bar and getting me sat down and the crutches were a pain.'

She also said: 'Maybe I have been putting all my eggs in one basket. I hadn't realized how much my kind of life depended on everything going just right. You win – I might consider putting two eggs in another basket even when I'm better!'

So the test results are in

Looking at the reports from the test pilots and the air controllers, it is clear that everybody who tested *Five:Two For a New You* felt they got some benefits from it. I have found it particularly interesting to compare their experiences with those of the two air controllers.

Poor old Mel suffered one of those unexpected accidents that catch us all from time to time, but it really knocked her lifestyle for six. Both she and I were surprised that such a comparatively minor thing as a knee injury could make such a big difference to how she felt.

We agreed that she'd been making a big assumption in how she lived her life – the assumption that she would always be able to go at a million miles an hour. As long as Mel was one hundred per cent, then everything was fine, but when she wasn't, things became tougher.

Five:Two for a rainy day

It made me realize that one of the big plus points about this technique is that having things in balance gives you the flexibility and adaptability to react to the unexpected and take it on board. As Mel admitted, by putting her eggs all in one basket, she hadn't left herself any leeway in case things went off course. So Five:Two is like having five eggs in one basket, and two in another basket.

There follows some of the other benefits that the test pilots and the air controllers discovered.

Five:Two Benefits

❖ **Self-knowledge** Several people mentioned that doing Five:Two had given them a better understanding of the things that really matter to them personally, especially through filling in the Life Staircase.

❖ **Adaptability** Everybody found they could use the principles in lots of areas of their life to help them be flexible in how they dealt with issues.

❖ **Problem solving** For most of us, the use of Five:Two to solve problems was the biggest plus of all. I personally found that every time something came up I found hard to handle, I could apply the principle and reach a solution.

❖ **Positivity** Because Five:Two is so solution-oriented, we found it a really positive experience to use it. You could relax about things and deal with them logically and methodically.

❖ **Accessibility** It's easy to do! Steph especially appreciated that you don't have to devote every waking moment to it in order to get results.

That's what we think – now it's over to you:
go out and Five:Two!

Useful Websites

There's almost too much information out there to help us. It can be difficult to know which sources to trust and which to ignore – and which are downright wrong! Here are some of the best websites I discovered while I was researching this book:

1. Fitness

There are thousands of great fitness sites on the internet. You could start with your health provider website and enter your key word. Here are some others to try:

www.runnersworld.com – a really good website to motivate you with your running.

www.fetcheveryone.com – this site also doubles as a personal log book/blog/running community and will be great if you are just getting interested in fun runs and races.

www.nrpt.co.uk – the home of the National Register of Personal Trainers will help you find a reputable trainer.

www.outdoorswimmingsociety.com – lots of help getting started with outdoor swimming.

www.britishorienteering.org.uk – official website to begin the sport.

www.hhs.gov – US government health site.

2. Work/Life Balance

www.citizensadvice.org.uk – has been handing out free advice for a long time and is a good first stop for work-related issues.

www.adviceguide.org.uk/england/work – handy all-round advice site, but you need to be quite specific in how you use it.

www.acas.org.uk – this is the home site of the independent and impartial Advisory, Conciliation and Arbitration Service, where you can get advice on workplace issues including flexible work, sick pay, maternity leave etc.

3. Relationships

www.relate.org.uk– website for marriage and relationship counselling in the UK.

www.thecoupleconnection.net – US-based forum with lots of good links.

www.mindtools.com – lots of free information about communication techniques.

www.do-it.org.uk – website for volunteering, especially charity projects, useful for finding new activities.

www.doitforcharity.com – web kit for arranging fund-raising events.

4. Beat the Years

www.ageuk.org.uk – the main go-to site in the UK for ageing-related issues, but is not the most positive as it concentrates on the problems of ageing rather than the fun side.

www.saga.co.uk – more or less the opposite of AgeUK, as it is very up-beat and can-do.

www.ageing.ox.ac.uk – website of Oxford Institute of Ageing, one of the world's leading centres for the study of ageing, packed full of the latest research.

www.nia.nih.gov – National Institute for Aging USA.

www.snac.org/eng – Sweden has among the longest-lived populations in the world, and the Swedish National Study on Ageing and Care is one of the reasons why. This is the English version of their website.

www.kungsholmenproject.se – the website for a fascinating study (again in Sweden) into preventing loss of mental faculties in old age.

www.karolinska.se/en/ – another Swedish project into ageing, this one looks at how to increase life expectancy.

5. Partying and Social Media

www.drinkaware.co.uk – along with www.gambleaware. co.uk these sites are a helpful first place to look if you are beginning to suspect you might have a real problem.

www.talktofrank.com – one of the more reliable sites to visit to get started thinking about drugs issues. Be careful what terms you use on search engines, as they can lead you to dodgy sites promoting various substances.

www.videogameaddiction.co.uk – though not fully recognized as addictive, many gamers are beginning to be concerned about how much time and money they are spending on their hobby, so this website is something to check out.

6. Parenting

www.education.gov.uk – another major element of the main government website. Check out some of the websites under Work/Life Balance as well for help with maternity leave etc.

www.mumsnet.com – a must visit, if only to keep up with other mums.

www.familiesusa.org – for users of healthcare, especially parents and children.

7. Well-Being

www.mind.org.uk – home of one of Britain's leading mental health charities, the first place to go for advice and contacts.

www.rcpsych.ac.uk – the website of the Royal College of Psychiatrists, aimed mainly at professionals, but a good place to find new research and contacts.

www.mentalhealthfirstaid.org – help for those suffering mental health issues.

www.aa.org – website for Alcoholics Anonymous.

Index

If you enjoyed *Five:Two For a New You*,

you'll love …

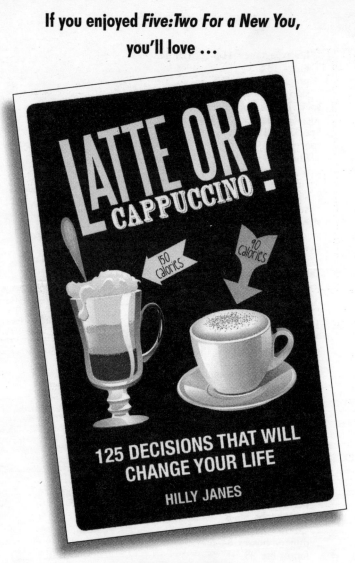

By **HILLY JANES**

ISBN 9781843175582   In paperback print format
ISBN 9781843178774   In ePub format
ISBN 9781843178767   In Mobipocket format